Medical Lives and Scientific Medicine
at Michigan, 1891–1969

Medical Lives and Scientific Medicine at Michigan, 1891–1969

Edited by Joel D. Howell

Ann Arbor

THE UNIVERSITY OF MICHIGAN PRESS

1996   1995   1994   1993   4   3   2   1

A CIP catalogue record for this book is available from the British Library.

Library of Congress Cataloging-in-Publication Data

Medical lives and scientific medicine at Michigan, 1891–1969 / edited
  by Joel D. Howell.
     p.   cm.
   Includes bibliographical references and index.
   ISBN 0-472-10465-9 (alk. paper)
   1. University of Michigan. Medical School—Biography. 2. Medical
research personnel—Michigan—Ann Arbor—Biography. 3. Physicians—
Michigan—Ann Arbor—Biography. 4. Medicine—Research—Michigan—
Ann Arbor—History.   I. Howell, Joel D.
   [DNLM: 1. University of Michigan. Medical School. 2. Education,
Medical—history—Michigan. 3. Physicians—biography. WZ 140 AM5
M489   1993]
R747.U6834M43   1993
610'.71'177435—dc20
DNLM/DLC
for Library of Congress   93-37106
                                                                    CIP

Acknowledgments

The editor expresses his appreciation to the three chairmen of the Department of Internal Medicine who supported this project. William N. Kelley, now Dean and Executive Vice President of the University of Pennsylvania Medical Center, initiated this project and gave it critical initial support. John Marshall, Interim Chairman at the University of Michigan and now Chairman of the Department of Internal Medicine at the University of Virginia, continued Dr. Kelley's support. Tadataka Yamada, the current Chair of the Department of Internal Medicine, supported the completion of the project.

The editor also thanks Terri Glazier for her administrative support of the project, and Clare Weipert for invaluable technical assistance.

Finally, the editor wishes to thank the faculty, students, staff, and patients of the University of Michigan Hospitals, all of whom made it possible for the individuals honored in this volume to do their work.

Contents

Introduction

Joel D. Howell

Medicine inevitably touches everyone. We all sometimes feel ill, wonder what is wrong, seek advice, and, often, recover our health. Our explanatory models have changed over the years, as well as the ways in which we seek to improve our health. Perhaps the most dramatic change occurred around the end of the nineteenth century, for from the late nineteenth century through the first half of the twentieth century, American medicine underwent a series of dramatic transformations. Those transformations both shaped and were shaped by changes in American society and changes in American medical schools.

The education of an aspiring physician shifted from apprenticeship with a practicing physician to attendance at a medical school. Medical school training became longer—extending from one or two years to four years—and came to include not only listening to lectures and sitting for examinations but also doing experiments and participating in direct patient care.[1] Most important, scientific validity became the touchstone of excellent medicine for both patient and physician alike.[2] Medical science was embodied, in part, in new medical machines that were used both in the laboratory and at the bedside. Technologies like the X-ray machine and the electrocardiograph machine became central to medical research and a routine part of medical care, anticipated and expected by patients.

With these changes in medical care came changes in the context within which medical schools functioned. Faculty members were expected to produce original research. Medical schools acquired hospitals with university affiliations. Much of the scientific research that was done in the American university early in the twentieth century was carried out in the medical school. Growing larger and more com-

---

1. Kenneth M. Ludmerer, *Learning to Heal: The Development of American Medical Education* (New York: Basic Books, 1985).

2. John Harley Warner, "Science in Medicine," *OSIRIS*, 2d ser., 1 (1985): 37–58.

plex, hospitals began to care for the middle class as well as the poor.[3] Eventually medical campuses came to dominate financially the universities they had joined, although they often found themselves farther away from the intellectual life of the parent school.[4]

We know a great deal about these events in broad strokes. But change took place slowly and incrementally. Scientific and social forces had their effect on specific persons and institutions, at specific times, for specific reasons. Although understanding the fine structure of change at the local level would be valuable, we have few analytic studies of events occurring at specific institutions.[5]

The University of Michigan Medical School warrants historical attention for at least two reasons. First, it provides historians with a glimpse of an area of the country that has been relatively overlooked. Most works on the history of American medicine have studied people and institutions on the East Coast. But medical practice eventually became a profession that defined itself as scientific because such a conception was widely shared.[6] The process of change may have been different in different regions of the country. Such prototypical private institutions as Johns Hopkins, the University of Pennsylvania, and the Rockefeller Institute were all located in large, established cities along the Eastern seaboard. The University of Michigan, a large state institution in a younger, smaller midwestern town, may present a different picture.[7]

3. Charles E. Rosenberg, *The Care of Strangers: The Rise of America's Hospital System* (New York: Basic Books, 1987).

4. Rosemary Stevens, *In Sickness and in Wealth: American Hospitals in the Twentieth Century* (New York: Basic Books, 1989).

5. George Washington Corner, *The Rockefeller Institute, 1901–1953: Origins and Growth* (New York: Rockefeller Institute Press, 1964); A. McGehee Harvey, Gert H. Brieger, Susan L. Abrams, and Victor A. McKusick, *A Model of Its Kind*, vol. 1: *A Centennial History of Medicine at Johns Hopkins* (Baltimore: Johns Hopkins University Press, 1989).

6. I refer here to medicine as practiced by regular M.D.'s, physicians who were trained to practice orthodox medicine. Other systems of medicine, such as homeopathy, chiropractic, and osteopathy, may have had less influence and power precisely because they failed to establish themselves as "scientific" as defined by orthodox university faculty.

7. Historians exploring science and medicine in a regional context outside the northeast have mostly looked at the American South. For introductions to this aspect of regional study, see Todd L. Savitt and James Harvey Young, eds., *Disease and Distinctiveness in the American South* (Knoxville: University of Tennessee Press, 1988); Ronald L. Numbers and Todd L. Savitt, eds., *Science and Medicine in the Old South* (Baton

Second, the University of Michigan has played an important, albeit often underappreciated role in the history of American medicine.[8] The first medical school to own its own university hospital (1869), the first major medical school to admit women (1870), the model for the medical school portrayed in Sinclair Lewis's *Arrowsmith* (1925), a leader in the early-twentieth-century reform of medical education, the University of Michigan was well recognized in the early and middle twentieth century as an institution of more than average influence.

Both the teaching and research programs at the University of Michigan have benefited greatly from excellent facilities for clinical care. The original University Hospital, which opened in 1869, was only a makeshift unit, a converted professorial residence, but it was the only university hospital in the United States. A new pavilion hospital served as the center of clinical instruction from 1874 to 1891.

Coincident with George Dock's arrival as Professor of Medicine in 1891, a new hospital opened on Catherine Street (fig. 1). Originally two main structures, one for the medical department and one for a

Rouge: Louisiana State University Press, 1989). For extension to the Midwest, see Thomas Bonner, *Medicine in Chicago, 1850–1950: A Chapter in the Social and Scientific Development of a City* (Urbana: University of Illinois Press, 1991); Leslie B. Arey, *Northwestern University Medical School, 1859–1959: A Pioneer in Educational Reform* (Evanston: Northwestern University, 1979); Leonard G. Wilson, *Medical Revolution in Minnesota: A History of the University of Minnesota Medical School* (St. Paul, Minn.: Midewiwin Press, 1989). Some have examined a regional midwestern identity: Madge E. Pickard and R. Carlyle Buley, *The Midwest Pioneer: His Ills, Cures, and Doctors* (Crawfordsville, Ind.: R. E. Banta, 1945). For recent attention to the Midwest at a statewide level, see Ronald L. Numbers and Judith Walzer Leavitt, eds., *Wisconsin Medicine: Historical Perspectives* (Madison: University of Wisconsin Press, 1981). Other works about specific states have been written; on Michigan, see C. B. Burr, ed., *Medical History of Michigan* (Minneapolis and St. Paul: Bruce Publishing Co., 1930).

8. Useful places to start for a history of medicine at the University of Michigan include Horace W. Davenport, *Physiology, 1850–1923: The View from Michigan* (Bethesda, Md.: American Physiological Society, 1982) and Horace W. Davenport, *Fifty Years of Medicine at The University of Michigan: 1891–1941* (Ann Arbor: University of Michigan Medical School, 1986). See also Richard M. Doolen, "The Founding of the University of Michigan Hospital: An Innovation in Medical Education," *Journal of Medical Education* 39 (1964): 50–57; Elizabeth Gaspar Brown, "Notes on the University Hospital: The Early Decades," *Michigan Quarterly Review* 3 (1964): 8–17; Wilfred B. Shaw, ed., *The University of Michigan: An Encyclopedic Survey*, 2 (Ann Arbor: University of Michigan Press, 1951); and a department-by-department survey in *Methods and Problems of Medical Education*, 18th ser. (New York: Rockefeller Foundation, 1930).

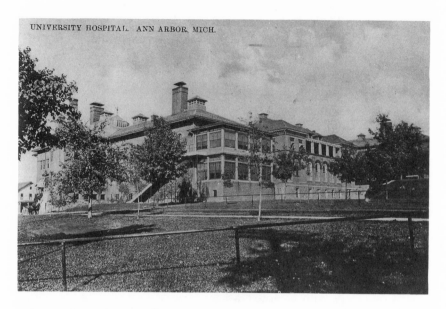

UNIVERSITY HOSPITAL. ANN ARBOR, MICH.

Fig. 1. The Catherine Street Hospital at the University of Michigan, circa 1902. (From a postcard in the editor's collection.)

homeopathic medical college, the facilities were augmented by a new homeopathic hospital (1900), a building for the care of children (1904), and one for the care of patients with diseases of the eyes and ears (1910). Other buildings were added for the care of patients with contagious diseases, diseases of the mind, and diseases of the skin, and for the treatment of pregnant women.

Starting in 1915, plans were made for a new university hospital to replace the scattered buildings on Catherine Street. Slowed by World War I and financial difficulties, the new hospital finally opened in August 1925 (fig. 2). It served well for over six decades, until another hospital opened in February 1986.

Following the 1986 move to a new hospital, the Department of Internal Medicine decided to name its inpatient services for historical figures at the University of Michigan. The names were selected based on a few defining characteristics. Because the services are based in the Department of Internal Medicine, all of the subjects either were faculty members in that department or, as in the case of Thomas Francis, did substantive work in areas associated with internal medi-

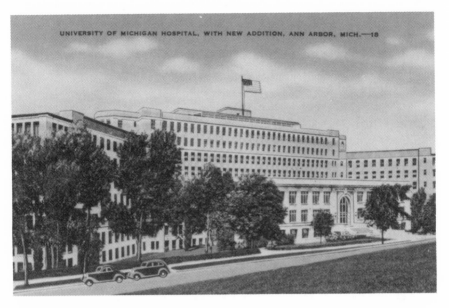

Fig. 2. The University Hospital at the University of Michigan, circa 1930. (From a postcard in the editor's collection.)

cine. These criteria left out several outstanding graduates of the medical school, such as William James Mayo, who graduated in 1883 and made the Mayo Clinic a center for excellence in medical practice, and Alice Hamilton, who graduated a decade later and helped define the field of industrial medicine.[9] Also, the department decided that no service would be named for persons still alive in 1986, when the service names were chosen. An internal medicine inpatient service was named after each person described in this book. The general medicine services are now named Dock, Francis, Hewlett, New-

---

9. Alice Hamilton provides an interesting contrast in Michigan's attitude toward women. On the one hand, Michigan admitted women long before any other major medical school; almost 30 percent of the students who graduated with Hamilton were women, and she fondly recalled her years in Ann Arbor. On the other hand, Dean Victor Vaughan made it quite clear, into the 1920s, that the University of Michigan Medical School was unwilling to employ a woman in a major professorial appointment. See Barbara Sicherman, *Alice Hamilton: A Life in Letters* (Cambridge, Mass.: Harvard University Press, 1984) and Bertha Van Hoosen, *Petticoat Surgeon* (Chicago: Pellegrini and Cudahy, 1947), 136–37.

burgh, and Sturgis, and the cardiology services are called the Wilson services.[10]

This volume does not present a broad synopsis of the history of medicine at the University of Michigan. Instead, the contributors take a biographical approach to some of the events at the University of Michigan from 1891, when George Dock assumed his position as head of the Department of Internal Medicine, to 1969, when Thomas Francis retired as chair of the Department of Epidemiology. Most of the figures described in this volume have thus far lacked serious analysis.

In the first chapter, Kenneth Ludmerer provides general background to the influence of the University of Michigan Medical School on the early-twentieth-century reform of American medical education. The dean of the Medical School, Victor Vaughan, maintained that research was an integral part of the faculty's academic mission (table 1). By the early 1890s, he had gathered together the strongest scientific medical faculty in the country. Ludmerer describes how Michigan became one of the first American medical schools to reform the curriculum, to replace lecture and demonstration by laboratory and clerkship, and to teach students how to acquire new knowledge throughout their career. The clinical clerkship at Michigan, introduced by George Dock in 1899, took advantage of the university-owned hospital and Dock's own enlightened approach to produce a clinical teaching program that became a model for other medical schools across the country (table 2).

The next six chapters trace the careers of a diverse group of physicians who contributed their services to science and medicine at the University of Michigan and their accomplishments to American medicine in general. Several themes run through these essays, including the nature of medical research, the reasons why each person remained at or left the University of Michigan, changing requirements for research support, the importance of the world wars, innovation in medical technology, and shifting boundaries within medicine.

---

10. Almost all of the chapters in this book were first presented as papers at the weekly Grand Rounds conferences of the Department of Internal Medicine at the University of Michigan. Alexander Leaf's reminiscences were delivered at a luncheon following the Grand Rounds.

American physicians in the late nineteenth century often sought advanced training in Germany.[11] Dock, Albion Hewlett, and L. H. Newburgh were among the thousands to take that journey. The three, however, returned with very different ideas about how to do medical research. Dock, trained in the nineteenth-century tradition of anatomic-pathologic correlation, saw research not as experiment, but as the careful compilation of clinical findings and the correlation of those findings with pathological anatomy. An active clinician, he based his research and teaching on the care of patients. Hewlett, Dock's successor as chairman of the Department of Internal Medicine, saw experimental physiology as the basic research tool. He wanted clinicians and basic scientists to work together on a regular basis. His vision of experimentation extended beyond the confines of the physiology laboratory. Hewlett wanted to create a university hospital that would be a major center for clinical research, a place

TABLE 1. Deans, University of Michigan Medical School, 1891–1970

Victor C. Vaughan	1891–1921
Hugh Cabot	1921–30
Executive Committee	1930–33
Frederick G. Novy	1933–35
Albert C. Furstenberg	1935–59
William N. Hubbard	1959–70

TABLE 2. Directors and Chairs of the Department of Internal Medicine, 1891–1975

George Dock	1891–1908
Albion Walter Hewlett	1908–16
Nellis Barnes Foster	1916
Louis Harry Newburgh	1917–22
Louis Marshall Warfield	1922–25
Preston Manasseh Hickey	1925
James Deacon Bruce	1926–28
Cyrus Cressey Sturgis	1928–57
Paul S. Barker	1957–58
William D. Robinson	1958–75

11. Thomas Bonner, *American Doctors and German Universities: A Chapter in International Intellectual Relations, 1870–1914* (Lincoln: University of Nebraska Press, 1963).

where patients not only received the finest in medical care but also served as the subjects for faculty investigation. Interestingly, the next major leader of the department, Cyrus Sturgis, though initially attracted by the new, experimental style of research, eventually drifted back to older ideas of clinical observation. Sturgis did run a department, however, that supported two physicians—Newburgh and Frank Wilson—who did major experimental and theoretical investigation.

Newburgh had visited Germany near the end of that country's widespread appeal for American physicians, shortly before a combination of World War I and the rapid improvement in American laboratories made German universities no longer a necessary stop on the way to learning about scientific medicine. He brought back an experimental, quantitative style of research far removed from Dock's clinical observations. Both Newburgh and his colleague Wilson turned to basic scientific disciplines for their fundamental methodology, a familiar move in the 1990s, but one unusual in the early decades of the twentieth century. In so doing, they helped shift the focus of medical research from the careful observation of sick people to the elucidation of fundamental biological and physical mechanisms of health and disease, a shift that has profoundly influenced modern medicine. Francis also changed his research focus. He started his career as a research virologist at the laboratory bench, but he moved the idea of experimental science out into the community, using a more global, epidemiological approach.

Some of the subjects of these chapters, such as Wilson, spent most of their career at the University of Michigan. Some, such as Dock and Hewlett, left their mark at Michigan en route to opportunities elsewhere. Their reasons for staying or leaving tell us much about what they thought important. Both Dock and Hewlett left Michigan at least partly because of inadequate laboratory facilities, though the meaning of the "laboratory" was different for each. For Dock, the laboratory was a place for students to be taught clinical pathology. For Hewlett, the laboratory was a place not only for clinical examinations but also for experimentation. For others, the institution provided a reason to found an entire career. Starting in 1925, Wilson enjoyed a new hospital designed in part to satisfy his needs. A new research institute helped entice Sturgis to come to Ann Arbor.

As the qualifications for academic status shifted from primarily clinical excellence and teaching expertise to scientific research accomplishments, research support became a major issue. Wilson and Newburgh were supported by the Rackham Fund, a private research fund at the University of Michigan that provided funds for investigative work in an era when other sources of support were essentially nonexistent. The University of Michigan tried to help its researchers by providing titles and time. Newburgh was named a "Professor of Clinical Investigation" in 1922, and henceforth had ample time protected to carry out his investigations. Francis was able to use University of Michigan students as experimental subjects for his work on influenza vaccine during World War II.

The two World Wars not only changed medical practice but provided the opportunity for productive, long-lived relationships. During World War I, both Sturgis and Wilson made important acquaintances with professional colleagues on the opposite side of the Atlantic while studying the elusive disease known as "soldier's heart." Later, Sturgis was forced to deal with the upheaval caused by World War II, as the manpower requirements of the U.S. armed forces greatly reduced the number of people available for work in the hospital. During World War II, as head of the Armed Forces Epidemiological Board's Commission on Influenza, Francis acquired broad powers and responsibilities, and he learned how to organize large-scale clinical trials. After World War II, Sturgis faced a new world of research paid for by the rise in available National Institutes of Health funding, a new world that had much to do with structural changes produced by the war.[12] Here, his older research values restricted his ability to pursue suddenly available federal research funds, funds primarily intended for basic research, rather than the clinical observations with which Sturgis felt most comfortable.

Twentieth-century medicine has become enamored of medical technology. Newburgh pursued his research agenda using a large calorimeter, a complicated device in which research subjects lived for months while Newburgh carefully measured their intake and outgo. Wilson spent most of his career melding mathematical theory with the technology of the electrocardiogram, and applying both to clinical practice. Some modern critics claim that an invention truly succeeds when we no longer see it as an invention, but as merely part of the

12. Daniel M. Fox, "The Politics of the NIH Extramural Program, 1937–1950," *Journal of the History of Medicine and Allied Sciences* 42 (1987): 447–66.

everyday world. Using this criterion, Wilson's ideas were certainly successful. Now taken for granted, his innovations became the basis for most of what is now the standard electrocardiograph tracing. Although "technology" is sometimes thought of as referring only to physical artifacts, it can also refer to activities or processes, as well as to the underlying knowledge for those processes.[13] Used in the broader sense, Francis's work with large-scale clinical studies, with the Army trials, and later with the Salk vaccine field trials, helped develop a new technology for the evaluation of community interventions.

Boundaries between different areas of medicine changed greatly during the twentieth century. Wilson, Newburgh, and Francis also helped redefine fields of medicine. Wilson popularized electrocardiography at a time when the term *cardiology* usually implied an interest in public health, not medical technology. Most people who wished to study heart disease drew inspiration from voluntary health societies, particularly those created to address tuberculosis. They viewed machines as peripheral to their central vision.[14] Wilson's study of the electrocardiogram provided the physical and intellectual tools necessary for the device to become a part of routine care (not to mention popular fare in television and movies). His laboratory also provided a place for students and colleagues to study the new instrument before it was accepted as a part of medical care. Newburgh's lifework gives us a valuable insight into the field of "metabolism." Though the subject matter Newburgh studied is now subsumed under other areas such as endocrinology and nephrology, in the 1930s it was one of the three basic areas of internal medicine, along with cardiology and microbial disease. Metabolism in the 1930s represented a way of bringing science in its most rigorous form into medical research. Physicians looked to diet as a major element in the treatment of disease, and depended on researchers such as Newburgh for guidance in the best way to accomplish their aims scientifically. Francis moved from

---

13. "General Introduction," in Wiebe E. Bijker, Thomas P. Hughes, and Trevor Pinch, eds., *The Social Construction of Technological Systems* (Cambridge, Mass.: MIT Press, 1987), 3–4.

14. Joel D. Howell, "Heart and Minds: The Invention and Transformation of American Cardiology," in Russell C. Maulitz and Diana E. Long, eds., *Grand Rounds: One Hundred Years of Internal Medicine* (Philadelphia: University of Pennsylvania Press, 1988), 243–75.

virology and immunology to establish epidemiology as an activist, interdisciplinary field for the study of diseases that could not be ignored. In so doing, he moved his gaze back from the laboratory to the patient, but he viewed his patients in the community, not in the hospital. Although George Dock looked at patients individually, and Thomas Francis looked at them as part of a community, they shared a vision, along with the other subjects of this book, a vision of medicine as a field of inquiry that creates new knowledge, through whatever means, and then applies that knowledge to improve the lives of human beings.

Biographical history has recently fallen out of fashion. When biography has been attempted, hagiography and history have blurred even more in the history of medicine than in general history. Nonetheless, biography offers the historian certain advantages, particularly when attempting to meld the internal content of a field with its social context. As Thomas Hankins points out, the human mind is, in fact, the level at which "scientific, philosophical, social, and political ideas [are all] wrapped up in a single package."[15] Moreover, a biographical approach helps greatly in examining an institution. The subjects of these chapters all interacted with a specific institution that often aided their desires, but occasionally impeded them. The subjects' lives serve as biopsies of a period and a place, as focal points to illuminate the personal nature of medicine and to place it within an institutional setting.

---

15. Thomas L. Hankins, "In Defense of Biography: The Use of Biography in the History of Science," *History of Science* 17 (1979): 1–16.

The University of Michigan Medical School: A Tradition of Leadership

Kenneth M. Ludmerer

During the nineteenth century, being a medical student in America was easy. No one worried about admission to medical school, because entrance requirements were lower than they were for a good high school. Instruction was superficial and brief. The terms lasted only sixteen weeks, and after the second term the M.D. degree was automatically given, regardless of a student's academic performance. Teaching was by lecture alone. Thus, students were spared the onerous chore of attending laboratories, clinics, and hospital wards. Indeed, except for the enterprising and affluent few who would bribe patients into submitting to an examination, students would often graduate without ever having touched a patient.

If this mode of medical teaching seems foreign in the 1990s, the organization and structure of the medical school are equally unrecognizable. In the post-Civil War era, the typical faculty consisted of seven or eight instructors. The schools were owned by the professors, who operated them for profit. For that reason, medical schools were called "proprietary schools." Medical teaching was a part-time activity, a side business to one's private practice. Since laboratories and hospital facilities were not utilized in medical education, only modest resources were needed to run a medical school. A second floor above a corner drug store would do; a school that had a building of its own was richly endowed. Very few schools had university affiliations or were connected with teaching hospitals, and medical research was almost nonexistent.

American medical education has changed dramatically in the twentieth century. Medical training has ceased to be a casual and superficial experience. Quite the contrary—it has become arduous, long, and demanding. Students are no longer taught by lectures alone. Instead, through laboratory instruction and clinical clerkships, they are made active participants in their own learning process. The schools—with their immense plants, sophisticated laboratories, capacious teaching hospitals, and large, full-time faculties—have become factories for the production of well-trained doctors and the pursuit of medical research. American medical education, once subservient to European medical education, has become the best in the world.

The maturation of American medical education was a complex process, one that spanned two continents and occurred over three-quarters of a century.[1] At the root of this transformation were broad forces that affected every institution of medical education: the revolution in experimental medicine of the middle and late nineteenth century; the cadre of American doctors who traveled to Europe to learn laboratory methods; the emergence of the modern university, which ultimately provided scientific medical schools a home in America; the development of a system of mass public education; the country's enormous expansion of wealth in the nineteenth century; and the emergence of a tradition of philanthropy that eventually made medicine its most-favored beneficiary.

But the story involves much more than broad social and scientific forces; it involves people and individual schools and hospitals as well. It is here that the University of Michigan Medical School played a crucial but often overlooked role. The school pioneered three of the most important areas of educational reform: the introduction of the modern curriculum; the promotion of medical research; and the development of the clinical clerkship. With the sole exception of the Johns Hopkins School of Medicine, no medical school in the country

---

1. On the evolution of America's present system of medical education, see Kenneth M. Ludmerer, *Learning to Heal: The Development of American Medical Education* (New York: Basic Books, 1985). Other helpful works on the history of American medical, education include William F. Norwood, *Medical Education in the United States before the Civil War* (Philadelphia: University of Pennsylvania Press, 1944); Martin Kaufman: *American Medical Education: The Formative Years, 1765–1910* (Westport, Conn.: Greenwood Press, 1976); Ronald L. Numbers, ed., *The Education of American Physicians: Historical Essays* (Berkeley: University of California Press, 1980); and William G. Rothstein, *American Medical Schools and the Practice of Medicine: A History* (New York: Oxford University Press, 1987).

served as a more-potent role model in shaping our nation's present system of medical education.

Curricular Reforms

In the early 1870s, the University of Michigan Medical School, although somewhat better than many American medical schools of the period, stood in desperate need of reform.[2] Admission was open to anyone who could pay the fees and demonstrate the barest familiarity with the English language. In 1871, only 14 of the school's 350 medical students held college degrees.[3] The curriculum consisted of two six-month terms of lectures, the second the same as the first. Instruction was almost wholly didactic. The main teaching device was the lecture, given before the entire student body assembled in a large amphitheater. Students endured six to eight hours of lectures daily, supplemented by textbook readings and occasional classroom recitation exercises. The anatomy course provided the opportunity for dissection, but the other scientific subjects were taught without the use of laboratories. Practical experience was provided in none of the clinical subjects. Students would graduate without having attended a delivery, without having witnessed an operation, and often without having examined a patient. All emphasis was on committing to memory the onerous details of the lectures. Some members of the faculty did wish to upgrade standards, but they feared that most prospective students would enroll instead at other schools with easier requirements.[4]

In 1877, however, the school extended its annual session from six months to nine, the first of a series of reforms that immediately placed the school in the vanguard of medical education. This was followed in 1880 by the introduction of a three-year, graded course (which ordered courses in a logical sequence—the basic science courses preceding pathology and therapeutics, and the scientific courses preceding the clinical work) and in 1890 by the introduction of a required fourth year. In the late 1870s, the school also began to

---

2. For an overview of the development of the medical school, see Horace W. Davenport, *Fifty Years of Medicine at The University of Michigan 1891–1941* (Ann Arbor: University of Michigan Medical School, 1986).

3. University of Michigan, *President's Annual Report* (1872), 12.

4. University of Michigan, *President's Annual Report* (1876), 11–12.

emphasize the scientific subjects and practical rather than didactic forms of instruction. Prior to 1877, instruction was primarily by lecture and demonstration; indeed, only two microscopes could be found in the entire school. By 1880, however, all students were receiving laboratory instruction in every scientific subject, with particularly extensive opportunities being provided in anatomy, chemistry, and physiology.[5]

Conditions were crowded; in 1878 there were 175 chemistry desks for 297 students, and many had to double up.[6] Nevertheless, teaching had taken on a genuine scientific form. These improvements were not undertaken without trepidation, for the faculty continued to worry that students might flock to schools with less-exacting standards. Yet after each reform, enrollment held.[7] What is especially noteworthy about these changes is that Michigan was only the second medical school in the country to embark on a program of reform. Previously, only Harvard Medical School in 1871 had undertaken a systematic effort to make its medical instruction more scientific and practical.[8]

The main instigators of the reforms were James B. Angell, the president of the University of Michigan, and Victor Vaughan, a biochemist and later dean of the medical school. Angell, one of the great first-generation university presidents, involved himself in every phase of the university's activities and guided Michigan's development into a major university. The first twenty years of his leadership (1871–91) saw an increase in the number of courses in the undergraduate college from 57 to 378; the introduction of modern languages, science, engineering, and laboratories; the adaptation of the German seminar; the promotion of independent study and research; the introduction and expansion of the elective system; the substitution of voluntary for compulsory attendance at chapel prayer; and the

---

5. Wilfred B. Shaw, ed., *The University of Michigan: An Encyclopedic Survey* (Ann Arbor: University of Michigan Press, 1942), 2:797; folder, "Reports of various departments of the Medical School regarding the work completed during the years, 1880–1882," box 72, University of Michigan Medical School Collection, Michigan Historical Collections, Bentley Historical Library, University of Michigan, Ann Arbor.

6. University of Michigan, *President's Annual Report* (1878), 13.

7. University of Michigan, *President's Annual Report* (1883), 13; *President's Annual Report* (1890), 90; and *President's Annual Report* (1891), 16.

8. Ludmerer, *Learning to Heal*, 47–63.

establishment of increased requirements for admission.[9] During the same period, Angell strove to invigorate all of the university's professional schools, which he felt should catch the "spirit" of university life.[10]

Angell's agent at the medical school was Vaughan, genial, relaxed, and soft-spoken, but tireless and indomitable in his mission to elevate standards of medical education. A veteran of German laboratory study—he had spent a year with Robert Koch learning the new science of bacteriology—Vaughan was determined to reshape the medical school into a center of advanced teaching and research. The task at Michigan was not easy, for the school was handicapped by geographic remoteness and the lack of even barely adequate hospital facilities. In addition, the senior member of the medical faculty, Alonzo B. Palmer—a spokesman of what Vaughan later termed the "old" rather than the "new" medicine—bitterly opposed Vaughan's first nominee to the faculty, the German-trained physiologist Henry Sewall.[11] Nevertheless, Vaughan persisted, appointing not only Sewall but also a group of eminent medical scientists who had gained experience in Germany: Franklin Mall in anatomy, John J. Abel and Arthur Cushny in pharmacology, William Howell and Warren Lombard in physiology, Paul Freer in chemistry, and Frederick Novy in bacteriology. By the early 1890s, Michigan had become, in the opinion of many, the strongest scientific medical school in the country. Vaughan proudly reminded readers in his autobiography that, of the original eight full professors of the Johns Hopkins Medical School in 1893, four had Michigan degrees and two were taken directly from the Michigan faculty.[12]

By the turn of the century, the quality of Michigan's medical teaching had reached world class and provided a model for other American medical schools to follow. Consider, for instance, the superb physiology courses offered by Warren Lombard starting in 1902. Each student, working with a partner, performed thirty-six experiments. Students would spend each afternoon from 1:00 to 4:30 in the laboratory, studying such phenomena as the extensibility and elastic-

9. University of Michigan, *President's Annual Report* (1891), 27–29.
10. University of Michigan, *President's Annual Report* (1882), 9.
11. Victor C. Vaughan, *A Doctor's Memories* (Indianapolis: Bobbs-Merrill, 1926), 199, 210–11.
12. Ibid., 223.

ity of frog muscle, the contractions of nonstriated muscle, the reaction time for sound, and the measurement of circulation, cardiac output, blood pressure, and respiration in mammals, usually rabbits or dogs.[13] Even the best university-affiliated medical schools of this period, in contrast, seldom offered laboratory instruction of this caliber, and many of the proprietary schools offered no laboratory work in physiology at all.

Of all the curricular changes Michigan introduced in the late nineteenth century, the most important by far pertained to the methods by which medicine was taught. The faculty helped bring about a revolution in pedagogic style; the role of the student was changed from passive observer to active participant in the learning process. The expansion in scope of the scientific and clinical teaching was important, but more fundamental still was the replacement of the lecture and demonstration by the laboratory and clerkship. Lectures, wrote the sharp-tongued Mall, were a "slow and stupid method of instruction," an outright "absurdity." The student must learn instead through personal study so that "he is upon the stage, not in the audience."[14] Through the laboratory and the clerkship students could learn by doing, not by watching.

The Michigan faculty believed that medical schools should now be charged with a new mission: that of teaching how to acquire and interpret information. For this reason, the school in 1880 adopted a policy, soon adopted by many other medical schools, that deemphasized the purchase of textbooks for the library and endeavored instead to subscribe to every major medical journal of the world.[15] Old truths were not to go unchallenged, and the knowledge gained by doing and experiencing was to be valued far more highly than that

---

13. "University of Michigan Laboratory Course in Physiology, 1904–1905" [mimeographed copy], folder 51, box 2, Warren Plimpton Lombard Papers, Michigan Historical Collections.

14. Franklin P. Mall, "The Anatomical Course and Laboratory of The Johns Hopkins University," *Bulletin of the Johns Hopkins Hospital* 7 (1896): 86. By 1896 Mall had left Michigan for Johns Hopkins, but the principles of education he advocated in Baltimore were the same as those he had earlier espoused in Ann Arbor.

15. Victor Vaughan, "The Medical School during the Administration of President Hutchins from October 1909 to June 1920" (typed report), n.d., box 8, University of Michigan Medical School Collection, Michigan Historical Collections. As late as 1876, the Michigan medical library subscribed to only one French and one German medical journal.

learned from the traditional authorities, the lectures and textbooks. It was now deemed more important for students to be able to understand biological phenomena and formulate judgments than to recite facts. This view of medical education stood in bold contrast to the prevailing view that the goal of medical education was to enforce the memorization of established facts and dogma. As George Dock admonished a group of clinical clerks at Michigan in 1907, every physician "must be able to recognize from what he has learned before new things, e.g., recognize unknown diseases by working them out from the diseases he has known before."[16] This could be done only if students developed the capacity to generalize from facts and principles already known.

If these views of the nature and purpose of medical education sound familiar to present-day observers, they are. The 1984 "GPEP" report of the Association of American Medical Colleges on training physicians for the twenty-first century incorporated these same ideals.[17] That study concluded that medical education should prepare students "to learn throughout their professional lives rather than simply to master current information and techniques." To accomplish this, students must be "active, independent learners and problem solvers rather than passive recipients of information."[18] Ideas in the writings and teachings of James Angell, Victor Vaughan, Franklin Mall, George Dock, and other members of Michigan's first scientific medical faculty have continued to guide medical educators in the United States from the late nineteenth century through the present.

The Promotion of Medical Research

If medical teaching suffered in post-Civil War America, medical research endured even greater obstacles. At no medical school in the 1870s did original research constitute a part of a faculty member's responsibilities. Professors lectured and tended to various administrative duties of the school. On their own time, they engaged in

---

16. "Clinical Notebooks of George Dock, 1899–1908," September 27, 1907, Michigan Historical Collections. See also session of September 30, 1904.

17. *Physicians for the Twenty-First Century. The GPEP Report. Report of the Panel on the General Professional Education of the Physician and College Preparation for Medicine* (Washington, D.C.: Association of American Medical Colleges, 1984).

18. Ibid., 9, 12.

private medical practice, performed consultations, and occasionally wrote textbooks. However, few faculty members felt they had the responsibility to promote the gathering of new knowledge. The rare medical professor who tried to conduct research, such as Charles E. Brown-Séquard at Harvard in the middle 1860s, did so on his own time and at his own expense.[19] No medical school supported or encouraged such work.

Nowhere were the difficulties encountered in pursuing medical investigation as a full-time activity more strikingly illustrated than in the case of S. Weir Mitchell, the founder of the American Physiological Society and the leading experimental physiologist of his generation. During the Civil War, Mitchell discovered that his interests lay with research rather than practice. He poignantly wrote his sister that he dreaded any distraction "removing me from the time or power to search for new truths that lie about me so thick."[20] Unfortunately, his colleagues did not share his enthusiasm for research. Twice at Jefferson Medical College (in 1863 and 1868) and once at the University of Pennsylvania (in 1868) Mitchell was denied the chair of physiology, despite having made vigorous efforts to secure the positions. Ironically, he had already established a reputation as a brilliant physiologist, having begun his pioneering experiments on snake venom that later became a foundation stone of modern immunology. One writer has found that Mitchell's success as an investigator actually impeded his receiving a chair.[21] In other words, Mitchell's prowess in physiological research stood in the way of his receiving a professorship of physiology at the two medical schools.

Mitchell was not alone in his inability to secure a position in full-time research and teaching. Particularly after the Civil War, as Americans started returning from postgraduate study in Germany, a

---

19. Brown-Séquard, born and trained in France, received the appointment of professor of physiology and pathology of the nervous system at Harvard Medical School in 1864. For three years, he conducted experimental studies in physiology, maintaining his laboratory at his own expense, until poor health forced him to resign his position. See C. E. Brown-Séquard to George Shattuck, March 17, 1865, and April 28, 1865, Dean's Office Files, Folder, "Letters to and from Professor Brown-Séquard," Countway Library, Harvard Medical School, Boston.

20. Quoted in Ernest Earnest, *S. Weir Mitchell: Novelist and Physician* (Philadelphia: University of Pennsylvania Press, 1950), 54.

21. Anna Robeson Burr, *Weir Mitchell: His Life and Letters* (New York: Duffield, 1929), 119.

whole generation of young, highly trained physicians encountered almost insurmountable obstacles to achieving their dreams of professional careers in medical research. Even in the 1870s and 1880s, laboratory positions were very scarce, and the few that did exist intimidated all but the hardiest spirits by their inadequate salaries, substandard facilities, decrepit sites, and, perhaps most important, lack of collegial support and encouragement. In 1878, William Welch, the famous Johns Hopkins pathologist and a beneficiary of European study, told his sister,

> I was often asked in Germany how it is that many good men who do well in Germany and show evident talent there are never heard of and never do any good work when they come back here. The answer is that there is no opportunity for, no appreciation of, no demand for that kind of work here.[22]

In this context, the appointment of Victor Vaughan to the deanship at Michigan in 1891 was epochal for the transformation not only of the medical school in Ann Arbor but of medical schools nationwide. From the start, influenced by his experiences studying medicine in Germany, he believed that the medical school should be a scientific school in distinction to a purely practical or clinical school. This meant that the basic sciences, in his words, should be "taught as a science and not as applicable to some practical problem"[23] and that persons selected for professorships must be productive scholars. "Medicine is a live, growing science," he wrote, "and no one is entitled to hold a chair in a . . . medical school who is not a contributor to the growth and development of his specialty."[24]

The development of medical research at Michigan, as in America, did not occur overnight. By today's standards, salaries were low, working conditions were arduous, and facilities were suboptimal. When John Jacob Abel was appointed America's first professor of pharmacology at the University of Michigan in 1890, he found that

22. Quoted in Simon Flexner and James T. Flexner, *William Henry Welch and the Heroic Age of American Medicine* (New York: Viking, 1941), 112–13.

23. Vaughan, *A Doctor's Memories*, 195.

24. Victor Vaughan, "The Functions of a State University Medical School" (unpublished manuscript, n.d.), 2, in file, "University of Michigan," Abraham Flexner Papers, Library of Congress, Washington, D.C.

he had to begin his new position without a laboratory of any kind. Using whatever space he could find, he had to borrow even such simple laboratory equipment as test tubes, flasks, and beakers.[25]

Nevertheless, the efforts of Vaughan and his supporters represented a major turning point in the development of American medical research. By the early 1890s, he had put together the strongest scientific medical faculty in the country. It was not by accident that Johns Hopkins raided Michigan for its first group of medical professors. Michigan's greatest contribution during these early years was not in the specific discoveries emanating from its faculty—important as some of these discoveries were—but its strong, unequivocal statement that original research was an essential function of the modern medical school. Good teaching alone would not suffice; medical schools had the duty to promote research as well. "In [medical] science we are still young," Vaughan explained, "but the time has come when we must cease to be mere followers of Germany and France."[26] This was a message that other medical schools heeded, and as a result, between 1890 and 1920, American medical research grew quickly to maturity and eventually assumed its present position of world leadership.[27]

Clinical Teaching

In the late nineteenth century, enormous improvements occurred in American medical education. Following the example of pioneering schools such as Michigan, medical schools across the country adopted four-year programs with nine-month terms, strengthened their requirements for admission, added all the new scientific and clinical subjects, and began giving their students some semblance of real laboratory instruction. The better schools also succeeded in establishing genuine relationships with a university, hired full-time faculty members, and began programs of medical research. By the early 1900s, the structure of the country's present system of medical education was firmly in place.[28]

---

25. "Copy of a Letter Written by Dr. John J. Abel to Dr. C. W. Edmunds, May 24, 1937, in Regard to His Early Work in Pharmacology at the University of Michigan," Michigan Historical Collections.

26. Vaughan, "The Functions of a State University Medical School," 3.

27. Ludmerer, *Learning to Heal*, 102–8, 123–38, 207–18.

28. Ibid., 72–122.

Nevertheless, medical education had not developed evenly. By 1910, the year of the famous Flexner Report, the strength of the country's medical schools had come to lie in the basic science instruction of the first two years. Equivalent progress in the clinical subjects had not occurred. Although the clinical courses provided students the latest knowledge, instruction remained primarily didactic, with limited opportunities for practical training. Very few medical students could be found caring for patients, which contrasted sharply with the scientific teaching and its use of laboratory instruction.

The dominant method of clinical instruction in the early 1900s was the section method of teaching. In this form of teaching, groups of students, as few as eight or ten per group at the better schools, would spend an hour or two a day, three to five days a week, examining patients in the hospital and following the progress of selected cases. With section teaching, students were closer to patients than ever before, and this certainly allowed for more personalized instruction than did lectures and textbook reading.

However, the section method contained an inherent flaw. It did not incorporate the principle of "learning by doing," as did laboratory instruction in the scientific courses. Bedside section teaching was much more effective than the didactic methods of early years, but it was still demonstrative. In that regard it was no different than the lecture and demonstration in the scientific subjects. This fact did not escape the eye of William Welch, who likened section teaching to

> the attempt to teach a subject like bacteriology by demonstrations of methods, cultures and microscopic slides instead of having the student make his own media, plant and cultivate the bacteria by his own hands, and follow and study from day to day with his own eyes the characters of the growing organisms.[29]

In section teaching, patients were cared for in the presence of students, but not by students. Students were passive observers, witnessing rather than participating in the medical work. Although frequently perceived as practical bedside instruction, section teaching was in reality little more than an illustrated lecture.

---

29. William Welch, "The Relation of the Hospital to Medical Education and Research," in William Welch, *Papers and Addresses* (Baltimore: Johns Hopkins University Press, 1920), 3: 135.

This pedagogic weakness was rectified only by the clerkship. Under this system, students not only received instruction in the hospital but became an active part of the hospital machinery. Rather than visiting the wards for an hour a day, students would be assigned four or six patients of their own and spend much of their day carrying out duties related to their patients' care.[30] This allowed students to experience rather than observe the conditions of medical practice. The famed internist William Osler of Johns Hopkins noted that all other forms of clinical instruction—the systematic lecture, the amphitheater clinic, the ward and dispensary classes—were but "bastard substitutes" for the clerkship.[31] For further progress, the clerkship had to be made available to every student.

The clerkship was struggling for one overriding reason: few medical schools had acquired control of teaching hospitals. Although most schools had access to clinical facilities, they were severely restricted in how they could use those facilities. Accordingly, instruction in the clinical departments was greatly hampered. Medical schools had no authority to decide whether students could work as clinical clerks, since permission of hospital boards was always required but seldom granted. Clinical professors were also handicapped in their own research, since they were often denied access to patients for purposes of clinical investigation. In addition, medical schools did not have the authority to appoint doctors to the staffs of their affiliated hospitals, which forced them to choose clinical faculty members from those who already had received a local hospital appointment; they did not have the liberty to select the best person who might be available anywhere.

Resistance to the clerkship was widespread among American hospitals of the period. Some of the best medical schools attempted to persuade their affiliated hospitals to see otherwise, but their efforts were unsuccessful. In 1906, the medical faculty of Columbia petitioned Bellevue Hospital for permission to introduce the clerkship,

---

30. For a description of the clerkship and its advantages over other methods of clinical teaching, see William Osler, "The Hospital as a College," in William Osler, *Aequanimitas with other Addresses to Medical Students, Nurses and Practitioners of Medicine,* 3d ed. (Philadelphia: Blakiston, 1932), 311–25.

31. William Osler, "The Fixed Period," in Osler, *Aequanimitas,* 389.

as did the faculty of Cornell in 1908.[32] Both requests were denied. Several times in the early 1900s, the medical staff of the New York Hospital asked the board of governors to permit students to be assigned cases in the wards, but each time the board refused.[33]

In the early 1890s, Harvard Medical School attempted to obtain a closer union with the Massachusetts General Hospital, but after four years of negotiations the hospital rejected the school's proposal.[34] In 1906, an editorial in the *Boston Medical and Surgical Journal* proclaimed a teaching hospital still to be "the greatest need of the Harvard Medical School."[35] During the first two decades of the century, the medical faculties of Yale, the University of Pittsburgh, the University of Minnesota, the University of Colorado, and the University of Southern California were also unable to convince their respective affiliated hospitals to become true teaching institutions.[36] Students often endured repeated indignities. In 1907, the trustees of the Peter Bent Brigham Hospital came within one vote of requiring students to enter and leave the hospital through a separate entrance.[37]

Tulane Medical School encountered similar obstacles in New Orleans, where the faculty's desire to introduce the clerkship was thwarted by its lack of authority in the administration of Charity Hospital. At Charity, the city's public hospital, teaching was unequivocally regarded as secondary in importance to care of the sick, creating conditions for clinical instruction that in the words of Tulane's professor of medicine were "absolutely rotten."[38] Tulane, which before the Civil War had been the jewel of the South in clinical teaching, had descended to the same level of mediocrity as schools elsewhere in the United States.

The greatest irony in the history of the clerkship involved

32. Faculty meeting minutes, May 14, 1906, College of Physicians and Surgeons, Office of the Dean, College of Physicians and Surgeons, Columbia University, New York; faculty meeting minutes, April 11, 1908, Cornell University Medical College, Medical Archives, New York Hospital–Cornell University Medical Center, New York.

33. Society of the New York Hospital, *Annual Report* (1910), 45.

34. James Clark White, file, "Committee on Improved Clinical Facilities, 1889–1892," Countway Library.

35. "The Need of a Hospital for the Harvard Medical School," *Boston Medical and Surgical Journal* 155 (1906): 352.

36. Ludmerer, *Learning to Heal*, 312, no. 49.

37. Trustee meeting minutes, September 6, 1907, Peter Bent Brigham Hospital, Administrative Office, Peter Bent Brigham Hospital, Boston.

38. Ludmerer, *Learning to Heal*, 312, n. 50.

Roosevelt Hospital in New York City. Established in 1863, it illustrated everything that was good about the nineteenth-century general hospital. Not only did it provide the most-modern clinical and technological services, but from the beginning it established an affiliation with the Columbia University School of Medicine (Physicians and Surgeons) and soon became the school's major clinical resource. The school regularly used the hospital's amphitheaters and clinics for teaching, and it was a popular choice among Columbia students for fourth-year electives and postgraduate internships and residencies.

However, when Samuel Lambert became dean of Columbia in 1905, he recognized that the relationship with Roosevelt was unsatisfactory for modern scientific teaching because the hospital did not permit the students to work as clinical clerks. Supported by his university president, Nicholas Murray Butler, Lambert requested the hospital to allow Columbia medical students to work as clinical clerks. As an added inducement, the medical school offered to raise $1,000,000 for a new surgical pavilion for the hospital if it would consent to do so. The hospital declined the offer. Columbia approached the hospital a second time in 1908 and a third time in 1910. Each time the hospital voted "no"; it did not want medical students in the wards as clinical clerks. Finally, after the third rejection, Columbia was able to negotiate such an arrangement with Presbyterian Hospital, and ultimately it was Presbyterian Hospital, not Roosevelt Hospital, that became the great international center of medical education and research in New York City. Roosevelt Hospital had the opportunity for greatness and threw that opportunity away.[39]

In this context, the contributions of the University of Michigan Medical School to clinical teaching were of monumental importance. When George Dock became professor of medicine in 1899, he introduced the clinical clerkship at University Hospital as the school's basic form of instruction in internal medicine. He could do so, whereas others had failed, because of his own enlightened views of clinical education and by virtue of the good fortune of having access to a teaching hospital under the medical school's direct control.

A highly sophisticated course, Michigan's clerkship rivaled that of Johns Hopkins, the only other school prior to 1910 to provide its students a consistently effective clinical experience. In this course,

---

39. Ibid., 160–65.

the students were given responsibility for patient care. At the start of each rotation, Dock would inform students that "the patient is under your care as part of your duties." He would instruct them "to follow up the case as long as the patient is in the hospital, seeing the patient at least once or twice a day." Students were required to make "daily observations and notes."[40] The clerkship at Michigan, as that at Johns Hopkins, quickly became a model for medical schools and hospitals across the country and helped usher in a new era of clinical teaching during World War I—an era that has lasted essentially unchanged through the present. In clinical teaching, as in curriculum reform and the promotion of research, the Michigan Medical School again served as one of the nation's pioneers.

Conclusion

The University of Michigan Medical School today enjoys a highly deserved reputation as one of the premier medical centers in the country. Not very well known, however, is the seminal role the school played in shaping America's system of medical education. With the sole exception of the Johns Hopkins School of Medicine, no school—even schools that are much older than the Michigan Medical School—can legitimately lay claim to such a long tradition of leadership, innovation, and influence.

---

40. Sessions of September 30, 1904 and September 27, 1907, "Clinical Notebooks of George Dock, 1899–1908," Michigan Historical Collections. For another detailed contemporary description of the sophisticated methods of clinical teaching employed at the University of Michigan, see C. L. Ford to the Editor of *Medical News*, n.d., folder, "Correspondence & Miscellaneous Material, 1902–1903 and Undated," box 72, University of Michigan Medical School Collection. See also Horace W. Davenport, *Doctor Dock: Teaching and Learning Medicine at the Turn of the Century* (New Brunswick, N.J.: Rutgers University Press, 1987).

George Dock at Michigan, 1891–1908

Horace W. Davenport

When thirty-one-year-old George Dock arrived in Ann Arbor in the autumn of 1891 to be Michigan's professor of internal medicine, he had already demonstrated the characteristics he shared with his mentor, William Osler, a preeminent physician and teacher of medicine. Those were insatiable curiosity about everything pertaining to medicine and a consciousness of the obligation to raise medical students and physicians to his own level of knowledge and practice.

In 1869 the University of Michigan converted one of the houses on North University Avenue, which had been built for a professor, into a dormitory for patients to be demonstrated or operated upon before the medical students in the medical building on East University Avenue. That is the basis of Michigan's claim to have had the first university-owned hospital in the country. In 1879 a pavilion hospital of 60 beds based on the Civil War hospital plan was added to the house. It was used for surgical patients, and it was scheduled to be torn down whenever it became hopelessly contaminated. An eye-and-ear ward was attached in 1881, in such a position that it blocked light from the pavilion hospital's operating room.

Consequently, when George Dock arrived he found no medical patients available for teaching purposes. He recruited Aldred Scott Warthin, a recent medical graduate, to be his assistant, and with the help of local clergymen they gathered enough patients to begin teaching.

From the time the medical school opened in 1850, there had been agitation to move the school, or at least clinical instruction, to Detroit where there would be more patients available than in Ann Arbor and more lucrative practices for the professors. The definitive decision to keep the school in Ann Arbor was made in 1879 by President James

B. Angell and the board of regents, and the two professors most vehemently opposed to the decision were dismissed. The Michigan Legislature appropriated $50,000 to build the University Hospital, and it was under construction when George Dock arrived. President Angell, reacting to the problems caused by having the pavilion hospital in the middle of the central campus, insisted that the new hospital be as far away as possible from the rest of the university, and it was constructed on Catherine Street, about a third of a mile distant (fig. 1). The Palmer Ward for children, who were cared for by internists until 1920, was added in 1903. By then Dock had about 140 beds for adult medical and pediatric patients.

As the reputation of the medical school spread, patients were referred from all over Michigan and surrounding states. There was, for example, a young black girl with tuberculosis sent from Gary, Indiana. Ann Arbor's population was less than 20,000, but the hospital beds were full and the outpatient clinic was crowded. In 1908, the year Dock left Michigan, the hospital had about 4,500 patient visits a year, and 1,967 inpatients (table 3).[1] Only three American university hospitals had more patients, and those were in large cities: Baltimore and Philadelphia. All Michigan patients, with the exception of university students, were, at least in theory, indigent, and all were in-

TABLE 3. Beds and Inpatients in Ten American University Hospitals in 1908

Hospital	Number of Beds		Patients in 1908	
	Total	Teaching	Total	Teaching
Johns Hopkins	353	288	4,609	3,845
Jefferson	346	286	5,044	3,680
Pennsylvania	344		4,342	2,856
Michigan	230 (270)*	230	1,967	1,967
Medico-Chirurgical		104	1,990	1,624
Iowa	135 (185)*	100	1,536	1,298
Virginia	100	75	1,300	950
California	78	70	822	660
Dartmouth	36	20	785	550
Colorado	40	30	300	150

Source: From A. W. Hewlett, *Physician and Surgeon* 31 (1909): 481–91.
* Numbers in parentheses includes additional beds under construction.

---

1. A. W. Hewlett, "The Relation of Hospital to Medical Schools in the United States," *Physician and Surgeon* 31 (1909):481–91.

cluded in teaching. Dock and some of his colleagues repeatedly frustrated Dean Victor Vaughan's attempts to move the clinical years to Detroit in search of a large patient population and, incidentally, more-lucrative private practice. Dock thought that thorough study of a few patients was preferable to cursory study of many patients in a large municipal hospital.

George Dock had been born in New Hope, Pennsylvania, on April 1, 1860, and after obtaining a good classical education at the University of Pennsylvania he entered the university's medical school in 1881. In Dock's time, the medical curriculum was three years long. There was a good anatomical laboratory, and Dock's demonstrator in surgical anatomy was C. B. Nancrede, later his colleague as professor of surgery at Michigan. Otherwise, there were lectures and demonstrations, but there was little hands-on laboratory work. The school did not have enough microscopes for the pathology course until after Dock had graduated. The school's catalog said that the students in their senior year had nine hours of work a week on the wards of the new University Hospital, but Dock found otherwise. Teaching of medicine was largely by lecture, and William Pepper, Jr., was particularly eloquent, being able to pass off a patient with jaundice for one with pernicious anemia if the latter were unavailable.[2] That did not satisfy Dock, and he told his Michigan students,

> I remember, for example, if an interesting patient was brought into the clinic, enterprising students would afterwards waylay him and by main strength or a small bribe get him to submit to an examination, but men got the title of doctor of medicine, with many elaborations in Latin, without having to handle a sick man.

When he graduated from medical school in 1884, Dock took a step unusual for those days: he interned for a year in a Catholic hospital in Philadelphia. The nurses were German nuns, and Dock learned conversational German from them in preparation for a trip to Europe. He also learned a great deal of clinical medicine, and at Michigan he often cited his hospital experiences. When he instructed Michigan students on how to obtain permission for an autopsy he

---

2. H. Cushing, *The Life of Sir William Osler*, 2 vols. (London: Oxford University Press, 1925), 1:284–85.

said that prejudice against an autopsy was not a Catholic but an Irish-Catholic phenomenon. When the family hesitated in the hospital, a word from a nun or a priest would hasten permission.

Dock studied in Austria and Germany in 1885–87, and he often told stories to Michigan students about Rudolph Virchow's dislike of bacteriology or how patients in a German military hospital had to stand at attention when an officer entered the ward. He spent the winter semester of 1885 in Leipzig working on microscopic pathology under Karl Huber, and he attended five autopsies every morning except Sunday.[3] Characteristically, he made a note that George Gruebler of Leipzig was a source of dyes, and he bought them from Gruebler when he had his own clinical pathology laboratory at Michigan.

The next spring, Dock took a six-week course in bacteriology from Arnold Becker, who had studied under Robert Koch. In the summer of 1886, Dock went to Berlin to work under Albert Fränkel in the Charité Hospital clinic of Ernst von Leyden. There Dock learned German methods of treating tuberculosis and the rules governing admission of tuberculous patients to German hospitals. Dock attended Carl Gerhardt's clinic and took courses in acute infections from Paul Guttman and in clinical pathology from E. Litten. He also attended Virchow's course in gross and microscopic pathological anatomy, given between 7:00 A.M. and 9:00 A.M. three times a week. He then did more clinical work in Vienna, and he continued to study pathology under Arnold Paltauf. Dock concluded his formal studies with a six-week course under Carl Weigert in Frankfurt. Dock's comments to Michigan medical students show that he informally studied German methods of physical therapy and that he visited the Dresden veterinary school to learn about intestinal parasites.

In Philadelphia a game of medical musical chairs left the chair of clinical medicine vacant, and the University of Pennsylvania recruited thirty-five-year-old William Osler to fill it. It is characteristic of Dock's passion for knowledge of medicine that, busy though he was as an intern, he sought out Osler to become Osler's disciple and then friend. Later Dock made "braindusting" trips with Osler, and he once accompanied Osler on a visit to Boerhaave's house in Ley-

---

3. G. Dock, "Clinical Pathology in the Eighties and Nineties," *Am. J. Clin. Path.*, 16 (1946): 671–80.

den. Dock and Osler corresponded regularly until the last year of Osler's life. Somehow Dock found time to follow Osler on the wards and to the autopsy room in Old Blockley, and after his German experience and his work in clinical pathology at the University of Pennsylvania, Dock was ready to assume a professorship of pathology in Texas in 1888 and the professorship of medicine at Michigan in 1891.

Dock shared Osler's love of old medical books, and he began to collect them on his own. On July 12, 1911, he and Osler attended an auction at Sotheby's in London where prices quickly rose out of their reach. Nevertheless, Dock did accumulate a substantial number of rare books in his long life, and when he died he left his collection to the library of the Los Angeles County Medical Association. Regrettably, the librarian failed to record which books had been Dock's, and it is now impossible to identify Dock's books in the library's catalog of rare books.

In 1907 Dock published a long article on John of Gaddesden's *Rosa Anglica*, whose purpose was to record the location of copies of the first edition of the book printed in Padua in 1492.[4] Dock's own copy was the 1502 Venice edition. *Rosa Anglica* has been called "a farrago of nonsense," but it does contain about forty words in Latin that influenced the care of smallpox patients into the twentieth century. Dock translated them:

> Let scarlet be taken and let him who is suffering from small pox be entirely wrapped in it or in some other red cloth. Thus I did when the son of the illustrious King of England suffered from small pox. I took care that everything about the couch should be red and his cure was perfectly effected, for he was restored to health without a trace of pocks.

In Ann Arbor, Dock explained to his students that he did not use red light in treatment of smallpox as practiced by Niels Finsen.[5]

Dock's love of books extended to the practical matter of a working library. When he came to Michigan, he found that the medical library had only sixty-one medical periodicals, of which only one was complete. Dean Vaughan made Dock chairman of the library commit-

4. G. Dock, "Printed Editions of the Rosa Anglica of John of Gaddesden," *Janus* 12 (1907): 425–35.
5. N. R. Finsen, *Phototherapy* (London: Edward Arnold, 1901).

tee and gave him the entire budget for journals and books. Dock worked quickly, and by 1895 he had completed all journals already in the library. When he started new subscriptions he bought a full set of back numbers. The result was that by 1905, the library contained 13,455 bound volumes and 226 journals, of which 99 were complete. The Michigan student who wants to consult Theodor Schwann's paper describing the discovery of pepsin published in the 1836 volume of *Archiv für Anatomie und Physiologie* or Adolf Kussmaul's paper describing the first use of the stomach tube published in the 1869 volume of *Archiv für klinische Medizin* will find them in the library because of Dock's efforts.

Dock encouraged medical students to improve their education by systematic reading in books and in domestic and foreign journals, and he gave them references to the latest article on how to observe the tracheal tug in aortic aneurysm or to a book on how to treat arthritis. He himself was always au courant. The patient at a diagnostic clinic on October 25, 1904, complained about the hospital food; it was tasteless. Dock said that he had ordered the food prepared without salt, as treatment for the patient's edema.

A quick search in the medical library showed me that Dock had been reading a series of papers published by Fernand Widal in a French journal in 1903. Dock had marked the entries for Widal in the index.[6] Widal had fed 10 grams of sodium chloride a day to patients with Bright's disease until they had pulmonary edema, anasarca, and epileptiform convulsions. The patients recovered when Widal withdrew the salt. Dock understood the relation between salt retention and water retention, and he explained to the students the principle underlying treatment of edema by salt restriction. The fact that Dock could order a salt-restricted diet shows that he had a competent dietician and an obedient cook in the hospital kitchen.

In Philadelphia, William Osler and John Herr Musser had each contributed $50 to equip a clinical laboratory in the University Hospital, and when Dock was in Germany he was asked to suggest how it should be furnished. Dock's inventory of sterilizers, autoclave, glassware, dyes, and microtome was approved by Carl Weigert. On return

---

6. [F.] Widal and [A.] Lemierre, "Pathogénie de certains oedèms brightiques: action du chlorure de sodium ingéré," *Bull. mem. Soc. méd. hôpit. Paris,* 3.s., 20 (1903):678–99.

to Philadelphia, Dock was put in charge of the laboratory, and Osler testified it was a busy place.

Dock established the same kind of laboratory in Ann Arbor, and by the time he left in 1908 he had earned the reputation of being the best clinical pathologist in the country. James Rae Arneill, who was Dock's assistant until 1903, published a 244-page manual of clinical diagnosis and urinalysis that describes the full range of equipment and methods Dock used in qualitative and quantitative examination of blood, gastric contents, sputum, feces, and urine.[7] Dock kept a culture of typhoid bacilli going, and he used the Widal flocculation test to confirm or disprove his diagnosis of typhoid fever. In 1905 Dock said he had done many thousands of gastric analyses, but because in other instances he used numbers carelessly, it is probable that he did fewer. Dock gave test meals, and he used a stomach tube to recover gastric contents which he titrated for free and total acid. He did not rely on a single meal for evidence of achlorhydria, which he thought was pathognomonic of cancer of the stomach.

Dock's laboratory was in his private office (fig. 3), but his assistants used it as well. Students could use it if they were assigned special tasks such as measuring daily the amount of sugar in the urine of a diabetic patient undergoing the prolonged test of glucose tolerance. Dock taught hematology, and he required his students to do red blood cell counts and differential white cell counts. Microscopes were always available in the clinic, and Dock had his students examine urinary casts and seek evidence of worms by examining the stool. Dock regretted that all students could not be taught methods of clinical pathology because there was no general laboratory for students' use. The basic science departments had student laboratories whose quality ranged from adequate in pharmacology to first class in anatomy, bacteriology, and physiology, but they were on the central campus far from the Catherine Street hospital.

No laboratories of any kind had been included in the hospital when it was built. Eventually, a small building was constructed for the hospital superintendent's office, and space freed in the hospital was used for a laboratory. Nevertheless, laboratories remained inadequate, and when A. W. Hewlett, Dock's successor, obtained an elec-

---

7. J. R. Arneill, *Clinical Diagnosis and Urinalysis* (Philadelphia: Lea Brothers and Co., 1905).

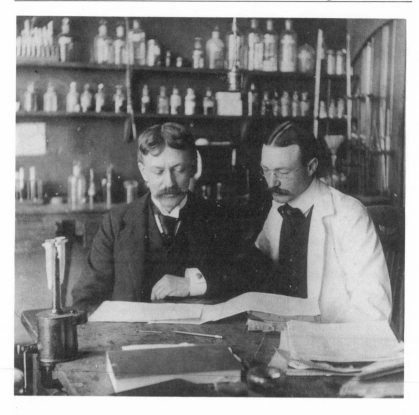

Fig. 3. George Dock and his assistant, James Arneill, in Dock's office-laboratory

trocardiograph it had to be housed in a closet under a stairway. There were no laboratories whatever for teaching, and Dock wanted one in which all students in their clinical years could have bench space and use of equipment kept in order by a full-time assistant. He repeatedly asked the university authorities to provide the laboratory, and in early 1908 he circulated a letter to his clinical colleagues asking their help. He did not get what he wanted, and that is one of the reasons he left Ann Arbor in the summer of 1908 for Tulane, where there was an excellent teaching laboratory for clinical pathology.

George Dock's son, William Dock, said that his father was "a sound, patient and not inspiring teacher until one decides to imitate his thorough and broad approach." George Dock was certainly a bad lecturer if a good lecturer is one who succinctly tells medical students what they are expected to know for an examination. Even when he was discussing a particular patient with a particular complaint, he was wildly discursive. For example, when Dock was talking about the self-limiting nature of pneumonia, he told students he had been raised in the heroic school of treatment and that by application of 9 × 5 to 12 × 18 inch poultices to both sides of the chest he had drawn "literally quarts of serum." They never did any good, and a "poultice has never shortened the disease by a minute." Then he described the controlled clinical trial that had shown that bleeding, salivation, and tartar emetic had produced no better result than no treatment at all. Then Dock said some doctors prescribed whiskey, because they thought whiskey strengthens the lungs. That led to a digression on the use of red pepper as a treatment of delirium tremens. On other occasions, Dock interrupted himself to cite Tolstoy's opinion that he could improve on Shakespeare, to say that false modesty in the clinic was as bad as putting skirts on statues in the Vatican, or to describe the Russian method of dealing with body lice.

Dock demonstrated his "thorough and broad approach" when he taught physical examination. One way he did that was to give a diagnostic clinic for senior students every Tuesday and Friday afternoon. For eight years, Dock engaged a stenographer to take down every word she could hear. He eventually donated the stenographic typescript, in sixteen volumes and totaling more than 6,800 pages, to the Michigan Historical Collections, and it is now in the Bentley Historical Library.[8]

Dock gave his clinics in an amphitheater of the Catherine Street Hospital, where students sat on tiers of remarkably uncomfortable seats (fig. 4). Years later Reuben Peterson, the professor of obstetrics and gynecology who used the same room, wrote:

[The seats] were simply terrible and every one of the clinical professors used to pity the students as they writhed on those seats. Dr. George Dock . . . was touched by the suffering of the poor medical students as he talked to them. When he concluded his lecture and turned to leave the amphitheater he remarked, "If after I leave this room you should tear those seats up, it would

---

8. H. W. Davenport, *Doctor Dock; Teaching and Learning Medicine at the Turn of the Century* (New Brunswick, N.J.: Rutgers University Press, 1987).

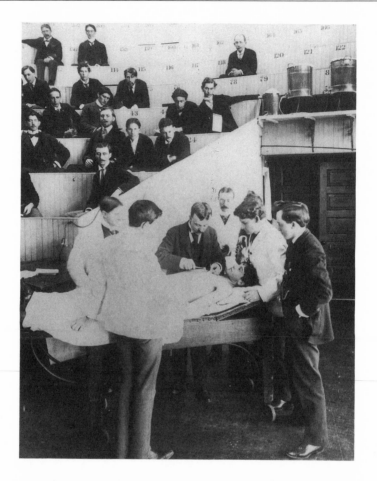

Fig. 4. George Dock purportedly examining a patient in one of his diagnostic clinics. James Arneill is standing behind Dock's left shoulder. The patient is wearing street shoes, and, in view of Dock's insistence that patients be completely exposed, it is obvious that a medical student posed as the patient for the sake of the picture.

grieve me terribly." The minute he left the students demolished those seats so that there was only kindling wood remaining.

The Regents fined the students a dollar each and reprimanded Dock.

Dock said that almost any medical problem could be solved through a thorough physical examination, and in his diagnostic clin-

ics he made his students do thorough examinations under his So-
cratic guidance (fig. 5). He did the same with students on the wards,
and in addition he had a number of specially competent students
acting as interns. He drove them all hard, and he expected them to
live up to his own high standards. When Alice Hamilton was a student in 1892–93, she was one of Dock's special students. She was
afraid of him, and she was wounded by Dock's scorn when she did
not know the life cycle of a fungus. Later, when Alice Hamilton
returned to Ann Arbor for a while, she wondered why she had been
so afraid of George Dock. It is clear that Dock was no antifeminist,
for he treated women students just as he treated the men, with the
exception that he always addressed them as Miss or Mrs. So-and-So
rather than by their last names alone. Dock corrected the students'
Latin and their spelling of English, and he was aware that his sharp
tongue and blasphemous remarks sometimes wounded his colleagues as well as his students.

At the time Dock taught at Michigan, the medical profession was
divided between those who, like Dock, had gone to good medical
schools and had on their own continued to improve their knowledge
and skill, and those ignorant doctors who had bought their degrees
from proprietary schools.

Dock was always polite to what he named "those so-called doctors," but in their absence he held them up as bad examples to his
students. Once, for instance, he related how he had overheard four
middle-aged doctors agreeing that no one had ever heard fetal heart
sounds and that the teachers who had told them about the sounds
were lying. Nine years after Dock left Michigan, his successor once
removed, Nellis B. Foster, had the duty of running a training school
for young physicians joining the army, and he was horrified to discover that only the graduates of a very few Class A medical schools
were capable of making a correct diagnosis. The others could not
differentiate between a diastolic and a systolic murmur, could not
tell the difference between pleural effusion and pneumonia, could
not recognize meningitis or diphtheria, and had never given antise-
rum.

Dock used the study of arthritis to teach his students how to
behave, and he once spent more than an hour leading one student
through the examination of every joint of an arthritic patient. He said
that when a student went into practice he would probably encounter

876,

Friday, May 12th, 1905.

PATIENTS: Carpenter (Hector), Mrs. Gibson (G. H. Lewis).
SECTION: Signor, Taylor, Thomas, Urquhart, Van den Berg.

Dr. We can pick out those who are neither lovers of music or base ball.

CARPENTER: Dr. Van den Berg, what do you think of this man? S. He looks sick. Dr. How does he look sick? S. His cheeks are slightly flushed and his eyes look rather bad. Dr. And what else? S. He is listless. Dr. What else do you notice about him? I think there is another thing that you ought to see. You have to be able to see it easily because when you see it at home it is usually in the alcove if there is an alcove about the house and the alcove is usually darkened so as to keep the air out as well as the light. S. I think there is cyanosis. Dr. That is the idea. There is cyanosis in his nose and it seems to me a little in his ears and lips and if we look at his hands we see a little in his nails, don't we? Otherwise there isn't anything so very striking about all that we can see of him now, is there? Let's see his tongue. Do you think there is anything abnormal about it? S. Why the terminal papillæ show very plainly. Dr. What else is there about it? How about the coating? He has a scanty but rather striking looking coat; that is the sort of a tongue that

Fig. 5. A page of the typescript of the stenographic record of George Dock's teaching. The comment about music refers to the fact that the third concert of the May Festival was given that afternoon.

an arthritic patient who had been given up by all the other doctors in town. The patient probably would not be able to pay, but the new doctor should care for her anyway. "While every man should see that he gets his pay, if possible, yet it is not a good thing to put this in the foreground." Careful and prolonged treatment might do the patient good, and care for such a patient would get the new doctor more credit than a hundred cases of pneumonia or typhoid. Then Dock gave the students instructions about treatment and recommended the English translation of Beir's *Hyperämie als Heilmittel* that he had read in German.

Dock, like Osler, was a clinical observer, not a scientist, and had little interest in the fundamental mechanisms of disease. His virtues and limitations are well illustrated by his dealings with diseases of the thyroid gland. He was thoroughly familiar with hyperthyroidism, but he could do little for a patient with Graves' disease except to put the patient to bed with an ice-pack over his heart. He did treat hypothyroidism with desiccated thyroid gland. He ignored the significance of the observations in 1895 by Adolf Magnus-Levy that the rate of oxygen consumption is elevated in hyperthyroidism and reduced in hypothyroidism and that both return to normal when treatment is effective.[9] Dock thought the method for measuring oxygen consumption was too complicated to be useful, not knowing that Warren Lombard, Michigan's professor of physiology, had invented a simple method of doing it.

Within a few weeks of Dock's arrival in Michigan, he saw more goiters than he had ever seen in Philadelphia or Galveston, for Michigan was a region in which goiters were endemic. Dock visited the Upper Peninsula and the northern parts of the Lower Peninsula where goiter was particularly prevalent. Fifty-two doctors responded to his questionnaire, reporting 477 cases. When Dock examined farm animals, he found goiters in horses, dogs, calves, and lambs.[10] The week after Dock attended the Junior Hop in the Waterman Gymnasium on February 14, 1908, he told his students:

> In fact, in this part of the country [a small goiter] has no anomaly because from my studies in the gymnasium at certain important functions of the year when people kindly prepare this part of their anatomy for inspection by doctors and others, I have found that 95 per cent of young girls have swellings like this.

---

9. A. Magnus-Levy, "Ueber den resparatischen Gaswechsel unter dem Einfluss der Thyroideas sowie unter veschiedenen pathologogische Zustäanden," *Ber. klin. Wochenschr.* 32 (1895):650–52.

10. G. Dock, "Goitre in Michigan." *Trans. Assoc. Am. Physicians* 10 (1895):101–6.

Dock went on to tell the students that

> When Wharton first described the thyroid in the 17th century,
> the only function he could imagine for it was that God had put
> it in the neck to improve the appearance of the neck which other-
> wise would have been made up of lines. He looked upon it as a
> pleasing piece of gallantry on the part of the Creator to make a
> more beautiful race.

For the sake of effect, Dock ignored the fact that Thomas Wharton
had proposed three other uses: to remove overflow of humors from
the recurrent laryngeal nerve, to warm the cartilages of the trachea,
and to lubricate the larynx. Dock knew the association of drinking
water with endemic goiter. He thought Michigan well water might
contain a toxin, and he advised patients to boil their water. As for
treatment, Dock found dried thyroid efficacious.

Dock's failure to draw a conclusion between the efficacy of dried
thyroid and the gland's iodine content contrasts with the behavior
of David Marine when faced with the same facts. When Marine arrived in Cleveland, Ohio, on July 1, 1905, and walked to the Lakeside
Hospital, he found goiters in dogs he met on the street. He decided
at once to tackle the problem of goiter.[11] Dock knew as much as
Marine did, but it was Marine who put the facts together in a fruitful
hypothesis and did the necessary experiments.

In Dock's time, the fields of endocrinology and deficiency diseases were just beginning to be cultivated, and Dock knew as much
as anyone about the results that had already been attained. He wrote
reviews about the topics, but he did no work on them. The one
instance in which he might have made an important discovery, he
had bad luck. When he was in Galveston, just before coming to
Michigan, he had tried to demonstrate that mosquitoes transmit malaria. He failed, because the wrong species of mosquito lived around
Galveston. Otherwise, he might have anticipated Ronald Ross.

George Dock was a physician in the Osler tradition, but I think
we overestimate the importance of Oslerian therapeutic nihilism.
Dock was nihilistic in his care of patients with pneumonia, for he

---

11. J. Matovinovic, "David Marine (1880–1976): Nestor of Thyroidology," *Perspect. Biol. Med.* 21 (1978):565–89.

knew that controlled clinical trials had shown that bleeding was harmful and poultices useless. He might have given strychnine to strengthen the patient's heart, but Osler used similar therapies we now laugh at. The attitude of Osler and Dock might be more accurately, if crudely, expressed in the questions: "What's he got, and what can I do for him?"

Dock was a superb diagnostician, but after the diagnosis there was a lot to be done. Dock saw that it was done. For example, there were many patients with typhoid fever in the University Hospital. The course of the fever was well-known, and Dock insisted that the patients' temperature be taken regularly and accurately. A drop occurred as the patient recovered at the end of four weeks, but a sudden drop was a signal that perforation was beginning and that it was time to call the surgeon before peritonitis or bloody stools appeared. A patient with typhoid fever was put in a cold bath for fifteen minutes every two hours. This was a heavy task for nurses and medical students, but both Dock and Osler thought the 4 percent improvement in mortality was worth the trouble.

In the case of diabetes mellitus, there was the long and tedious process of attempting to measure the patient's glucose tolerance. When smallpox appeared, Dock mobilized the medical students for a mass vaccination program, what he called a "vaccination debauch," in Ann Arbor as well as in the hospital. Then there was the long-term care of the smallpox patient, which included frequent bathing with a dilute solution of mercuric chloride to reduce scarring. For the many tuberculous patients, there were the problems of nursing care, of prevention of cross-infection in the patient's family, and advice on long-term treatment at home or in the West. Above all, there was the campaign to teach medical students the necessity of early diagnosis of tuberculosis. Arthritis was another problem of long-term care, and Dock knew all about the German methods of physical therapy. He taught them to his students, and he tried to persuade them to use the methods when they were out in practice.

Dock wanted his students to reach his standards. Sometimes students neglected their duties, but if that were because they were overwhelmed by work on other services Dock excused them, saying they should never undertake more than they could handle. If students did not have a valid excuse, Dock reprimanded them, but in doing so he said they were harming themselves as well as their patients. If the student failed to help the nurse with the tedious and repetitious task of giving cold baths to a patient with typhoid fever, Dock said: "These tubs are not given to you as punishment, but as a privilege. . . . Anyone with eyes or even a rudimentary cortex can't spend fifteen minutes with a typhoid patient without learning something." On another occasion, when a student failed to observe a patient undergoing the test for possible tuberculosis, Dock gave him a long lecture on what the student ought to have seen. Dock ended by saying: "So you missed your chance and nobody else who has a similar opportunity should neglect it."

President Angell, who was growing old and arbitrary in 1908, told Dock he had heard Dock was thinking of taking a job at Tulane. Would Dock please make up his mind soon so that the University could go about looking for his successor? Dock did go to Tulane, but he stayed there only two years. Then he went to Washington University in St. Louis, where he was dean as well as professor of internal medicine. Dock did not like the medical school's adoption of a policy of hiring only full-time faculty, however, and after a few years he resigned to enter private practice in Pasadena, California. He died at the age of ninety-one.

Albion Walter Hewlett: Teacher, Clinician, Scientist, and Missionary for "Pathologic Physiology"

W. Bruce Fye

Though his tenure as professor of medicine at the University of Michigan was brief—from 1908 to 1916—Albion Walter Hewlett left his imprint on the institution (fig. 6). He sought to convince his colleagues and pupils that newer laboratory tests could be employed to the patient's advantage, and he continued the tradition of bedside instruction pioneered in America by his teacher William Osler and introduced at Michigan by his predecessor George Dock.

Hewlett entered medicine when advances in science were being incorporated into medical practice at an unprecedented rate. Between the time he entered medical school and his selection as professor of medicine at Michigan thirteen years later, X-rays were discovered, many clinically relevant bacteriological techniques were developed, the electrocardiogram was introduced into clinical practice, the sphygmomanometer was invented, the Wassermann test for the serological diagnosis of syphilis was introduced, tuberculin skin testing was developed, and several clinically useful biochemical tests were devised.[1] Hewlett appreciated the significance of these and other dramatic developments and urged their implementation at Michigan.

I thank the archivists of the Johns Hopkins Medical Institutions, Stanford University, and the University of Michigan for their assistance and for granting permission to incorporate manuscript materials from their collections into this article.

1. W. D. Foster, *A Short History of Clinical Pathology* (Edinburgh: E. & S. Livingstone, 1961). See also Stanley J. Reiser, *Medicine and the Reign of Technology* (Cambridge: Cambridge University Press, 1978) and Knud Faber, *Nosography: The Evolution of Clinical Medicine in Modern Times*, 2d ed. (New York: Paul B. Hoeber, 1930).

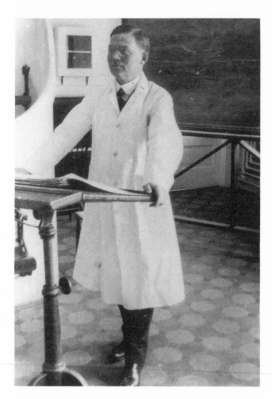

Fig. 6. Albion Walter Hewlett teaching a class

He also hoped to convince his colleagues and pupils to look at their patients' complaints in a new way. Symptoms, according to Hewlett, reflected deranged function or disordered physiology—a departure from the traditional view that structural abnormalities were the seat of most physical complaints.

Hewlett's lasting influence at Michigan, later at Stanford, and in American medicine is due largely to the general acceptance of his conviction that patients could be best served if a thoughtful clinical evaluation at the bedside or in the clinic were supplemented with selected laboratory tests. Today, we take this for granted. But it was Hewlett and some of his contemporaries in Europe and America that provided the proof that this approach was both efficient and effective.

Walter Hewlett was born on November 27, 1874, in Petaluma, California, about thirty miles north of San Francisco. He was the son of Frederick and Cleora Whitney Hewlett. Shortly after he was born, his family moved to San Francisco. As a young man, Hewlett attended the San Francisco Boys' High School and the University of California at Berkeley with Joseph Erlanger, who would win the Nobel Prize in physiology or medicine for his contributions to electrophysiology.[2] While a student at Berkeley, Hewlett learned of the new medical school at Johns Hopkins from Herbert Moffitt, a native of San Francisco who was in his senior year at the Harvard Medical School. Although his friend Erlanger entered Johns Hopkins, Hewlett remained in San Francisco and matriculated to Cooper Medical College.

Like many other American medical schools at the close of the nineteenth century, Cooper Medical College was in a state of flux when Hewlett enrolled there in 1895. The curriculum had just been extended to four years and a building that included "large and well-equipped laboratories for chemical, microscopical, pathological, bacteriological and physiological work" had just been completed.[3] Ray Lyman Wilbur, an instructor in physiology at Cooper when Hewlett was there, later recalled that the institution was then "undergoing a transition from the old-style commercial medical school to the modern scientific medical school." He characterized the large classes at Cooper as "made up of a rather unruly lot of Americans, varying all the way from boys who had just finished high school to others who had taught school or been in other positions for several years and then decided to study medicine."[4]

In 1895 there were more than 200 students enrolled in the school. In contrast, the new Johns Hopkins Medical School had fewer than half this many pupils—Erlanger's class numbered 33.[5] After completing one year at Cooper, Hewlett taught physics and chemistry at St.

2. See also A. McGehee Harvey, "Albion Walter Hewlett: Pioneer Clinical Physiologist," *Johns Hopkins Med. J.* 144 (1979): 202–14, and Joseph Erlanger, "A Physiologist Reminisces," *Annu. Rev. Physiol.* 26 (1964): 1–14. Additional biographical information was kindly provided by William Hewlett, Palo Alto, Calif.

3. *Cooper Medical College San Francisco, Annual Announcement Session of 1896* (San Francisco: W. A. Woodward & Co., 1896). See also Robert G. Whitfield, "Historical Development of the Stanford School of Medicine. A Thesis Submitted to the School of Education and the Committee on Graduate Study of Stanford University," 1949, Lane Medical Library, Stanford University Medical Center (hereafter referred to as Lane Library).

4. Edgar E. Robinson and Paul E. Carroll, *The Memoirs of Ray Lyman Wilbur, 1875–1949* (Stanford: Stanford University Press, 1960), 79, 82.

5. "Minutes of the Cooper Medical College," leaf 183, October 14, 1882–August 14, 1899, Lane Library. See also Alan M. Chesney, *The Johns Hopkins Hospital and the Johns Hopkins School of Medicine, A Chronicle*, vol. 2, *1893–1905* (Baltimore: Johns Hopkins University Press, 1958).

Matthew's School in San Mateo. He hoped to join Erlanger at Johns Hopkins, however, and applied for admission to the second-year class. He informed William H. Welch, the dean of the Johns Hopkins Medical School, that courses he had taken at the University of California and at Cooper justified his request for advanced standing. Moreover, Hewlett claimed that he had the highest average in his class of more than 50 at Cooper.

When the Hopkins faculty refused his request for admission to the second-year class, the young Californian wrote Welch again, this time enclosing testimonials from his professors at the University of California and Cooper Medical College. Joseph LeConte of the University of California told the Hopkins faculty that Hewlett "was one of the best students I ever had." Levi Lane, president of Cooper, described Hewlett as "a faithful, successful, and popular student." Hewlett's second letter to Welch was a seven-page essay lobbying for advanced standing. He closed by explaining, "to take a second year is for me out of the question principally for financial reasons." Hewlett's persistence paid off. His request for advanced standing was approved, and he entered the second-year class at Johns Hopkins in October 1897.[6]

Unprecedented opportunities for participation in research were available to Hopkins medical students in this era. Hewlett took advantage of this stimulating environment and, with Erlanger, studied the effects on absorption of surgically shortening the small intestines of dogs. This research, undertaken in William Howell's physiology laboratory during Hewlett's second year at Hopkins, resulted in Hewlett's first publication.[7] Following his graduation from Hopkins in 1900, he spent two years as an intern and resident on the medical service of the New York Hospital.

An experience that shaped Hewlett's career was eighteen months of study in Tübingen with Ludolf Krehl, a leading German

6. The relevant correspondence is Hewlett to Welch, January 11, 1897; Hewlett to Welch, March 22, 1897; Joseph LeConte to Professors of the Medical Department, February 25, 1897; Levi Lane [to Welch], February 26, 1897; and Welch's notes on his replies to Hewlett, January 18, 1897 and April 2, 1897, Alan M. Chesney Archives, Johns Hopkins Medical Institutions.

7. Joseph Erlanger and Albion Walter Hewlett, "A Study of the Metabolism in Dogs with Shortened Small Intestines," *Am. J. Physiol.* 6 (1901): 1–30.

medical scientist and physician.[8] Krehl was one of the first to encourage the study of abnormal function—pathologic physiology—in contrast to abnormal structure—pathologic anatomy—which was emphasized by Rudolph Virchow and his pupils.[9] Upon his return from Germany in 1903, Hewlett was appointed assistant in the medical clinic at Cooper Medical College, where the facilities for teaching and research had been dramatically improved. Oliver Jenkins came from Stanford University to teach physiology, and Ray Wilbur oversaw the equipping of a new physiological laboratory in 1898. This laboratory was equipped with apparatus for research as well as for demonstrations and laboratory exercises.[10]

Hewlett's interests were shifting from animal experiments to clinical research, however. Reflecting his enthusiasm for the new field of pathologic physiology, he translated Krehl's pioneering monograph on the subject, which had first appeared in 1893. Although Krehl's title was *Pathologische Physiologie*, Hewlett entitled his translation *The Principles of Clinical Pathology*, "to emphasize the fact that the book deals especially with the problems that confront the clinician."[11] Krehl sought to integrate clinical skills learned at the bedside with newer scientific approaches to the diagnosis of disease that relied on laboratory techniques. William Osler, one of Hewlett's professors at Johns Hopkins and America's leading physician, contributed an introduction to Hewlett's translation of Krehl's book. He praised the book for approaching disease as "a perversion of physiological function."

8. H. Dennig, "Zum 100. Geburtstag von Ludolf von Krehl," *Muench. Med. Wochenschr.* 103 (1961): 2489–93.

9. Russell C. Maulitz, "Pathologists, Clinicians, and the Role of Pathophysiology," in Gerald L. Geison, ed., *Physiology in the American Context, 1850–1940* (Bethesda: American Physiological Society, 1987), 209–35; Gerald L. Geison, "Divided We Stand: Physiologists and Clinicians in the American Context," in Morris J. Vogel and Charles E. Rosenberg, eds., *The Therapeutic Revolution: Essays in the Social History of American Medicine* (Philadelphia: University of Pennsylvania Press, 1979), 67–90; Winfield S. Hall, "Pathologic Physiology, A Neglected Field," *JAMA* 45 (1905): 1995–96; William G. MacCallum, "On the Teaching of Pathological Physiology," *Bull. Johns Hopkins Hosp.* 17 (1906): 251–54.

10. *Annual Announcement of the Cooper Medical College* (San Francisco: Cooper Medical College, 1898), 16.

11. Ludolf Krehl, *The Principles of Clinical Pathology, A Text-Book for Students and Physicians*, trans. Albion Walter Hewlett (Philadelphia: J. B. Lippincott, 1905), 3.

The main focus of Hewlett's research throughout his career was the cardiovascular system. This interest can be traced, in part, to Krehl, who published several papers on the heart and circulation and an important monograph on diseases of the myocardium, which George Dock translated into English.[12] Hewlett shared an interest in graphic methods for studying the circulation in man with Arthur Hirschfelder, whose father, Joseph Hirschfelder, was professor of medicine at Cooper Medical College when Hewlett was a student there. Like Hewlett, the younger Hirschfelder was a graduate of the Johns Hopkins Medical School and had studied in Germany. In 1904, they both were on the faculty at Cooper, but the following year Hirschfelder returned to Hopkins as director of the new physiological laboratory in the medical department.[13]

In 1906 Hewlett published a paper on paroxysmal tachycardia, the first of many he wrote on cardiac arrhythmias. James Mackenzie of Great Britain and Karel Wenckebach of Germany had made important observations on cardiac arrhythmias using a sphygmograph, and Hewlett used this approach in his early investigations of disorders of the heartbeat.[14] During the five years Hewlett was on the Cooper faculty, he published several papers on cardiac arrhythmias and conduction disturbances as well as a study of the effect of amyl nitrite on blood pressure and papers dealing with pancreatic enzymes.

Financial concerns at Cooper while Hewlett was there, however, led the officers of the school to restrict purchases of supplies and to seek other means of increasing the efficiency of their operation. The great San Francisco earthquake and fire in 1906 necessitated even harsher measures to reduce expenses at Cooper and at its clinical

---

12. Ludolf Krehl, *Die Erkrankungen des Herzmuskels und die Nervösen Herzkrankheiten* (Vienna: Alfred Hölder, 1901); Ludolf Krehl, "Diseases of the Myocardium and Nervous Diseases of the Heart," in George Dock, ed., *Diseases of the Heart* (Philadelphia: W. B. Saunders & Co., 1908), 421–763.

13. A. McGehee Harvey, "Arthur D. Hirschfelder—Johns Hopkins's First Fulltime Cardiologist," *Johns Hopkins Med. J.* 143 (1978): 129–39. See also Lewellys F. Barker, "The Organization of the Laboratories in the Medical Clinic of the Johns Hopkins Hospital," *Bull. Johns Hopkins Hosp.* 18 (1907): 193–98.

14. Albion Walter Hewlett, "Doubling of the Cardiac Rhythm and Its Relation to Paroxysmal Tachycardia," *JAMA* 46 (1906): 941–44; Albion Walter Hewlett, "Digitalis Heart Block," *JAMA* 48 (1907): 47–50; and Albion Walter Hewlett "The Interpretation of Positive Venous Pulse," *J. Med. Res.* 17 (1907): 119–36.

facility, the Lane Hospital.[15] In a report to the faculty four months after the disaster, Cooper's president informed his colleagues,

> From such calamities all enterprises pecuniary and beneficent as well as educational and social must necessarily suffer. In addition to this Cooper College has suffered serious damages to its buildings, making expensive repairs necessary, and so depleting its funds as to delay the institution of contemplated additions and improvements.[16]

Undoubtedly, Hewlett's clinical and research activities were affected by the disaster and its serious economic consequences for the medical college and hospital. As the city of San Francisco was recovering from the earthquake and fire, the directors of Cooper sought solutions for their financially troubled institution. They decided to deed the properties of the medical school to Leland Stanford Junior University, which had been founded in Palo Alto in 1885 and opened six years later. This union, which Cooper officials had considered for several years, took place on January 1, 1908.

Hewlett remained at Cooper Medical College only a few months after it was taken over by Stanford. It was already apparent that he was destined to be a leader in the new era of internal medicine— where the scientific physician trained in the laboratory as well as at the bedside would be the academic model and, according to the reformers of medical education, the most successful practitioner. Despite his youth, Hewlett's scientific contributions were already being acknowledged by other Americans who also sought to encourage clinical research and the new scientific medicine. In 1907 he was invited to join eight other physicians in establishing a society for clinical investigators. Samuel J. Meltzer, a New York physician with a strong background in experimental physiology, sought to form an organization for young physicians interested in research. Thus, Hewlett became a founding member of the American Society for the

---

15. See Minutes of July 1, 1905, April 27, 1906, and May 6, 1906, Cooper Medical College Directors Minutes, vol. 2, 1900–1905, Lane Library.

16. Minutes of August 13, 1906, Cooper Medical College Directors Minutes.

Advancement of Clinical Investigation, a group known familiarly as the "Young Turks."[17]

By 1908 Hewlett had been promoted to assistant professor at Cooper, where, with William Cheney, the professor of medicine, he was responsible for teaching the fourth-year students. The medical course consisted of lectures, discussion groups, and demonstrations in the dispensary. Compared with his experiences at Johns Hopkins, the New York Hospital, and in Germany, it is likely that Hewlett found Cooper rather confining in this era of uncertainty following the earthquake. When Abraham Flexner visited Cooper in 1909 he concluded that, from the standpoint of medical teaching, the organization of the Lane Hospital was "seriously defective." In his acerbic style, Flexner wrote, "The catalogue statement that the [Lane] hospital is a teaching hospital is hardly sustained by the facts."[18]

By the time Flexner visited Cooper Medical College, Hewlett had left the institution—a more promising opportunity had drawn him to the University of Michigan. At the turn of the century, Michigan's medical school was one of America's most progressive institutions for the training of physicians. The university could claim several leading medical researchers among its graduates when their chair of medicine became vacant in 1908. While a student at Johns Hopkins, Hewlett undoubtedly heard his professors talk about the midwestern university where several of them had received training. Franklin Mall, William Howell, and John J. Abel, professors of anatomy, physiology, and pharmacology, respectively, had all received degrees from or taught at Michigan. Henry Hurd, superintendent of the Johns Hopkins Hospital, received his undergraduate and medical degrees from Michigan as well. William Osler, Hewlett's professor of medicine at Hopkins, also held the medical program at Michigan in high regard. In 1908 he told his former resident George Dock, professor of medicine at Michigan, "You have worked the small farm

17. Allen R. Brainard, "History of the American Society for Clinical Investigation, 1909–1959," *J. Clin. Invest.* 38 (1959): 1784–1864; A. McGehee Harvey, *Science at the Bedside: Clinical Research in American Medicine, 1905–1945* (Baltimore: Johns Hopkins University Press, 1981).

18. Abraham Flexner, *Medical Education in the United States and Canada*, bull. no. 4 (New York: Carnegie Foundation for the Advancement of Teaching, 1910), 193–94.

at Ann Arbor to perfection. Bradford was speaking the other day of how gratified he was with the medical side of Ann Arbor."[19]

Dock, Michigan's professor of medicine since 1891, informed the university's president, James B. Angell, of his acceptance of the chair of medicine at Tulane University in July 1908.[20] Concern about the amount of clinical material available for medical teaching and practice in Ann Arbor, a town of 20,000, had led some on the faculty to urge a union with the Detroit Medical College. The debate became bitter and contributed to Dock's departure. Aldred S. Warthin, professor of pathology, had considered going to Tulane with Dock but decided to remain at Michigan. He informed Walter Sawyer, a Hillsdale physician and one of the university's regents,

> I have done this because I still believe in the School and in its future and think that with wise management, even if we can never compete with some of the great clinical centers, we can take the dignified and honorable position held by many of the smaller German Universities—where, after all, so much of the best German work has been done. It will all depend upon the character of the men that we get here to fill vacancies. What we need is men having the interest of the University at heart, and high ideals of work; and who are not tempted by the financial rewards of practice.[21]

Dock's resignation was anticipated, and the officers and faculty at Michigan hoped to secure Rufus Cole, an associate in medicine at Johns Hopkins, to succeed him. Cole visited Ann Arbor but turned down their offer when he was chosen as director of the new Rockefeller Hospital for Medical Research in New York. He informed

---

19. Osler to Dock, George Dock file, Osler Library, McGill University. See also Horace W. Davenport, *Fifty Years of Medicine at the University of Michigan, 1891–1941* (Ann Arbor: University of Michigan Medical School, 1986) and Kenneth M. Ludmerer, *Learning to Heal: The Development of American Medical Education* (New York: Basic Books, 1985).

20. George Dock to James B. Angell, July 31, 1908, University of Michigan Board of Regents Collection, box 3, September 1908 file, Michigan Historical Collections, Bentley Historical Library, University of Michigan, Ann Arbor (hereafter referred to as Bentley Library).

21. Warthin to Sawyer, July 31, 1908, in Walter Sawyer Papers, correspondence file, July 1908, Bentley Library.

President Angell, "It is with very great reluctance that I have given up the idea of casting my future there [Ann Arbor] and laboring under such pleasant circumstances and with such able colleagues."[22] When Michigan's medical dean Victor Vaughan informed Sawyer that Rufus Cole would not be coming to Ann Arbor, he reassured the regent, "We have several men on the string, and hope to have complete information concerning a few of them by the time the Board meets."

In his letter, Vaughan revealed his frustration with Dock:

The hospital here certainly needs improvement and revision. The work in Internal Medicine has fallen greatly behind. Both the late incumbent and his assistants greatly neglected the work last year, and we wish to revive and to get a man who will not be so pessimistic but will go to work in earnest and build up the work in that department. Whatever may be the ultimate result of clinical teaching in Detroit, you and I are certainly agreed that the clinic teaching here must be greatly improved, and there is no reason why it should not be. I think the Faculty is now a unit, perfectly harmonious and determined to pull together for the very best interest of the University.[23]

Rufus Cole urged the Michigan faculty to select Walter Hewlett for their chair of medicine. Hewlett had graduated from Johns Hopkins one year after Cole, and they were both charter members of the new society for clinical investigation. Michigan graduate Franklin Mall, now professor of anatomy at Johns Hopkins, informed Carl Huber, Michigan's anatomy professor, that Hewlett was "one of our very good men."[24] It is likely that Hewlett's special interest in physi-

---

22. Cole to Angell, August 17, 1908, James B. Angell correspondence, box 7, Bentley Library. Other correspondence regarding the Dock resignation and the Cole nomination is James B. Angell to Sawyer, July 31, 1908 and August 7, 1908; Vaughan to Sawyer, July 27, 1908, Sawyer Papers, box 1, correspondence file July 1908; and Franklin Mall to Carl Huber, July 17, 1908, Gotthelf Carl Huber Papers, Bentley Library. See also, Davenport, *Fifty Years of Medicine*, 221–23.

23. Vaughan to Sawyer, September 10, 1908, Walter Sawyer correspondence, September 1908, Bentley Library. See also Victor C. Vaughan, *A Doctor's Memories* (Indianapolis: Bobbs-Merrill, 1926).

24. Mall to Huber, August 24, 1908, Gotthelf Carl Huber Papers, Bentley Library.

ologic pathology was viewed as an asset as well—several members of the Michigan faculty believed in this new approach.[25]

Vaughan informed the Michigan regents that Hewlett had already had offers from Harvard and Tulane, that he had done admirable clinical research, and that his appointment would "give credit to the Medical Department." On behalf of the faculty, he urged them to select Hewlett for the medical chair, offering to share with them letters "from the most prominent men in Medicine in this country concerning the ability of Dr. Hewlett, and his fitness for the position."[26] Regent Sawyer moved that Hewlett be appointed professor of internal medicine and director of the clinical laboratory at a salary of $3,000, effective October 1, 1908.[27]

Vaughan telegraphed Hewlett, "Cole has written you concerning the chair of medicine in Michigan University. Would you accept same at $3000?"[28] Hewlett telegraphed his acceptance and wrote to James Angell,

> I wish to express to you my gratification at being appointed to the chair of internal medicine at the University of Michigan. I think that you have there the ideal university medical school, free from the distractions which necessarily occur in a large city. I realize my difficulty as a successor to George Dock but hope that I will fill the chair satisfactorily.[29]

At their meeting of October 19, 1908, the faculty of Cooper Medical College accepted Hewlett's resignation with regret and wished him well in his new position.[30] Franklin Mall told Carl Huber, "You have an excellent man in Hewlett, & he will do you honor. He is excellent in every respect."[31] Scottish pharmacologist Arthur Cushny, who had

---

25. Peyton Rous, "The Teaching of Physiological Pathology at the University of Michigan," *Bull. Johns Hopkins Hosp.* 19 (1908): 336–38.

26. Vaughan to Board of Regents, September 24, 1908, University of Michigan Board of Regents Collection, box 3, September 1908 file, Bentley Library.

27. *Proceedings of the Board of Regents* (Ann Arbor: University of Michigan, 1906–10), 354, Bentley Library.

28. Copy of telegram [September 28, 1908] in Medical Faculty Meeting Minutes, vol. 1907–10, leaf 411, Bentley Library.

29. Hewlett to Angell, October 1, 1908, James B. Angell correspondence file, box 7, Bentley Library.

30. Cooper Medical College medical faculty minutes, vol. 3, 99, Lane Library.

31. Mall to Huber, October 9, 1908, Gotthelf Carl Huber Papers, Bentley Library.

served on the Michigan faculty from 1893 to 1905, informed Huber, "I was very glad to hear you had got Hewlett at the U. of M. I fancy he is a very good man, from what of his work I have read and his line is more intelligible to me than Dock's."[32]

Of Hewlett's selection, his colleague Frank Wilson recalled,

> Hewlett was one of the first men appointed to the chair of medicine in an important medical school whose chief interest lay in the functional rather than in the structural aspects of disease—in pathologic physiology rather than in pathologic anatomy. He had a strong instinct for research, and his reputation rested more upon his attainments in the field of productive scholarship than upon his renown as a clinician.[33]

Dock's departure from, and Hewlett's arrival at, the University of Michigan were celebrated in a ceremony in the fall of 1908. An address by Reuben Peterson, professor of obstetrics and gynecology, and portraits of Dock and Hewlett appeared in the Michigan medical journal the *Physician and Surgeon* to mark the occasion. Peterson's laudatory remarks about Dock made it clear that Hewlett was following a man who was well liked at the university. But Peterson reassured his audience, "Men whose opinions carry great weight and who have had the best opportunities of judging Dr. Hewlett pronounce him the best young clinician in the country."[34]

Thus, Hewlett left California for Ann Arbor at the age of thirty-three to become professor of medicine at the University of Michigan. Teaching and clinical research were his main activities in Ann Arbor. When he arrived there, the third-year students were taught internal medicine by lectures and in the clinic, where they learned physical diagnosis and simple laboratory techniques for examining body fluids. Hewlett taught them the etiology, symptomatology, and physical

---

32. Cushny to Huber, January 3, 1909, Gotthelf Carl Huber Papers, Bentley Library.

33. Frank Wilson, "The Department of Internal Medicine. II. The Years 1908–27," in Wilfred Shaw, ed., *The University of Michigan: An Encyclopedic Survey* 2 (Ann Arbor: University of Michigan, 1951), 838–42.

34. Reuben Peterson, "Remarks at the Opening Exercises of the Department of Medicine and Surgery at the University of Michigan, upon the Resignation of George Dock, for 17 Years Professor of Medicine, and upon Albion Walter Hewlett, His Successor," *Physician and Surgeon* 30 (1908): 485–88.

signs of disease. Senior students learned the principles of differential diagnosis and treatment as well. For them, emphasis was on bedside teaching and hospital work. They were assigned patients admitted to the medical wards and were responsible for obtaining the admission history and performing the physical examination and routine laboratory tests.

Hewlett or one of his associates rounded daily with the students. His dedication to teaching is emphasized by his practice of rounding each Sunday morning with a select group of students who had a special interest in internal medicine. They followed patients throughout the year, not just during their assigned medical rotation. Hewlett also held weekly demonstration clinics and regular sessions devoted to newer diagnostic techniques. Medical teaching at Michigan reflected William Osler's influence on George Dock and Walter Hewlett as well as Hewlett's exposure to clinical teaching in Germany.[35]

When Hewlett joined the University of Michigan in 1908, the hospital facilities on Catherine Street comprised four main buildings containing more than two hundred beds. In addition there were two amphitheaters, clinical laboratories, and rooms for diagnostic and therapeutic X-rays.[36] The school's 1908 announcement noted that the University of Michigan Hospital was "instituted primarily for teaching purposes, as all who are admitted are utilized freely for instruction."[37] Hewlett was pleased with the university's commitment to teaching in its hospital—he felt this was the primary role of a university hospital.[38] In 1903 a spacious new laboratory and classroom building for the scientific branches of the medical curriculum had opened next to the old medical school building. The facilities at Michigan must have seemed quite satisfactory to Hewlett when he arrived there in 1908.

---

35. Osler's methods of teaching at Johns Hopkins when Hewlett was there are summarized in William Osler, "An Address on the Medical Clinic; a Retrospect and a Forecast," *Brit. Med. J.* 1 (1914): 10–16.

36. Reuben Peterson and Wilfred Shaw, "The University Hospital," in Shaw, *University of Michigan*, 2: 953–75. See also George Dock, "The University Hospital: Its Past, Present, and Future," *Michigan Alumnus* 9 (1903): 183–92.

37. *University of Michigan. Department of Medicine and Surgery. Annual Announcement, 1908–1909* (Ann Arbor: University of Michigan, 1908), 47.

38. C. de Nancrede, A. W. Hewlett, A. M. Barrett, "Report of the Committee on the Relation of the University Hospital to the Medical Profession," attached to leaf 505, Faculty Meeting Minutes, 1907–10, Bentley Library.

Valuable insight into Hewlett's attitudes toward medical education and health care is provided by an address he delivered shortly
after his arrival in Ann Arbor. He emphasized the dramatic changes
that were occurring in medical education in the United States. He
applauded the emergence of full-time careers in the medical sciences
that encouraged research and improved the quality of medical instruction. He looked forward to the expansion of the full-time system
to the clinical departments. Like other progressive medical educators
of the day, Hewlett attributed Germany's preeminence in medicine
to the emphasis placed on research in her universities and welcomed
the appearance of the same ethic in America.

Reflecting his conviction that the science and the art of medicine
should be closely integrated, Hewlett argued,

> In the thorough study of a disease, pathological, physiological,
> chemical, and bacteriological problems are frequently encoun-
> tered. The department of medicine needs the cooperation and
> assistance of the departments of pathology, physiology, physi-
> ological chemistry, and bacteriology. In a similar manner, the
> practical therapeutist is benefitted by contact with the scientific
> pharmacologist. The clinical departments should be given the
> benefits of the closest possible association with the scientific de-
> partments. The scientific men, in their turn, are often aided by
> this association and the constant reminder of the problems which
> confront the clinician often give a practical turn to their work.[39]

This address was delivered the year before Abraham Flexner
published his influential study of American medical education, sponsored by the Carnegie Foundation. Flexner was impressed by Michigan's medical school when he visited Ann Arbor in the spring of 1909
to collect information for his report. He observed that students were
taught the medical sciences in well-equipped laboratories, by men
who were "productive scientists as well as competent teachers."
Flexner applauded the fact that every patient in the university's hospital could be "used for purposes of instruction." In his opinion, the

---

39. Walter Albion Hewlett, "The Relation of Hospitals to Medical Schools in the
United States," *Physician and Surgeon* 31 (1909): 481–91; W. Bruce Fye, *The Development
of American Physiology: Scientific Medicine in the Nineteenth Century* (Baltimore: Johns
Hopkins University Press, 1987).

liberal policies of the school made up for the disadvantages of its small-town location: "The thoroughness and continuity with which the cases can be used to train the student in the technique of modern methods go far to offset defects due to limitations in their number and variety."[40]

Victor Vaughan, a member of the American Medical Association's Council on Medical Education and an ardent supporter of medical school reform, was enthusiastic about Flexner's project. Shortly after Flexner visited Ann Arbor, Vaughan informed Regent Walter Sawyer,

> Last Friday Dr. Flexner of the Carnegie Foundation spent the day here inspecting the Medical Department. He is inspecting all the medical schools in the United States. The Carnegie foundation will make a report upon medical education in this country, in England, France and Germany. I am sure that such a report will be of the greatest service to the profession and the better medical schools.[41]

Hewlett sought to make medical practice more scientific by teaching physiological principles and techniques that could be employed in the evaluation of patients. When electrocardiography was introduced into clinical practice in Europe, he quickly realized the potential of this technique. In 1909 he informed readers of the *Physician and Surgeon* of the important observations made with the instrument by Ewald Hering, a German pioneer of electrocardiography. Hewlett published his review the same year Alfred Cohn of New York brought the first electrocardiograph to America—and four years before Hewlett would acquire one for the University of Michigan. Hewlett was excited about the potential value of this new instrument and observed, rather prophetically, "It is not improbable that the electrocardiogram will ultimately permit of an early diagnosis of disease of the heart muscle."[42]

---

40. Flexner, *Medical Education*, 243–44.

41. Vaughan to Sawyer, April 8, 1909, Walter Sawyer Papers, April 1909, Bentley Library.

42. Albion Walter Hewlett, "The Clinical Value of the Electrocardiogram," *Physician and Surgeon* 31 (1909): 322–23. See also Frank Wilson, "The Heart Station," in Shaw, *University of Michigan*, 2: 988–89, and W. Bruce Fye, "The Delayed Diagnosis of Myocardial Infarction: It Took Half a Century!" *Circulation* 72 (1985): 262–71.

Hewlett's sophistication in, and contributions to, cardiovascular physiology led British cardiologist Thomas Lewis to select him as one of six coeditors of his new journal, *Heart,* which first appeared in 1909. They developed a friendship, and Lewis visited the Hewletts during a trip to America. Beginning in 1912, Hewlett offered an elective course in the clinical physiology of the circulation. This was limited to six junior students and dealt with disturbances of cardiac rhythm, the consequences of valvular lesions, the causes and effects of hypertension, pulmonary edema, and other subjects of clinical relevance. During his tenure at Michigan, Hewlett published several papers on cardiac arrhythmias and disorders of cardiac conduction, as well as papers that reflected his interest in the peripheral circulation and endocrine disorders.

Harry Hutchins succeeded James Angell as president of the University of Michigan in 1910, and Victor Vaughan prepared a report on the medical school for the new president. Hewlett contributed the section on internal medicine, in which he made a plea for more adequate clinical laboratory space and advocated the construction of a laboratory building on the hospital grounds. The increasing number of patients at the hospital and the growing reliance of physicians on diagnostic tests would further strain the laboratory which, according to Hewlett, also had insufficient space for teaching and research. In his review he made reference to the recently published Flexner report, in which the clinical material for instruction in internal medicine at the University of Michigan was characterized as only "fair." Hewlett reassured Hutchins, "Fortunately [the number of patients] has been increasing rapidly" and included a table showing that the number of patients in the hospital had nearly doubled during the preceding four years.[43]

Reflecting his growing recognition as a leader in the new field of pathologic physiology, Hewlett served as chairman of the section of pathology and physiology of the American Medical Association in 1913. At the annual meeting of the AMA held in Minneapolis that year, he delivered a paper entitled, "The Relation of Pathologic Physiology to Internal Medicine." In this address Hewlett revealed his

---

43. Albion Walter Hewlett, "Internal Medicine and Diseases of Children," in Victor C. Vaughan, "Report from the Department of Medicine & Surgery to the President [Harry B. Hutchins] of the University," in Harry Hutchins Papers, Report of the Medical School, box 20, 1910, 20–23, Bentley Library.

optimism about the development of effective therapies for medical disorders. He pointed to recent advances in knowledge of the pathophysiology of several diseases and to new therapeutic approaches that had produced effective therapy for malaria, syphilis, and some deficiency diseases. He also applauded the growing appreciation of the value of preventive medicine among American physicians and concerned citizens.

Pathologic physiology, "the science of disturbed function," provided a new approach to the diagnosis of disease and served as a scientific basis for therapy directed at correcting disturbances of function, much like surgery was aimed at curing structural abnormalities. The efforts of clinicians and scientists had to be merged if the full potential of the new scientific medicine was to be realized, however. Clinicians must have access to laboratories, and scientists had to stay in touch with the needs of physicians and patients.[44]

Victor Vaughan and the university's regents appreciated Hewlett's efforts. His salary was $4,000 in 1915, the highest salary of any medical faculty member at Michigan. But Vaughan explained that Hewlett devoted "practically all his time to his work." In other words, he had essentially no private practice. Two professors of surgery who were paid less than Hewlett received additional income from consultation fees. Vaughan argued against equal salaries for faculty members. He told the president of the University of Texas, "A man ought to be paid what he is worth and the salary should not be determined by the position which he holds." It is apparent that Vaughan thought Hewlett was worth a great deal to Michigan.[45]

Then, as now, academic physicians were often as much concerned with their facilities and staff as with their salaries, however. The facilities for Hewlett's department were, in fact, quite modest, and, eventually, he became frustrated with them. President Hutchins was informed in October 1915,

The hospital committee learned at its meeting this morning that Dr. A. W. Hewlett was considering accepting the Chair of Medi-

---

44. Albion Walter Hewlett, "The Relation of Pathologic Physiology to Internal Medicine," *JAMA* 61 (1913): 1583– 86.

45. Vaughan to W. J. Battle, March 23, 1916, in University of Michigan Medical School Collection, miscellaneous correspondence, box 32, July 1916, A–N, Bentley Library.

cine at the University of Minnesota. The Doctor gave as his reason for considering the appointment the fact that he had been
unable to secure here, proper facilities for establishing a clinical
and experimental laboratory. Inasmuch as the Hospital Committee feels that Dr. Hewlett's loss will be severely felt by this Medical School the Committee requests that his wishes be given favorable consideration.[46]

The following year, Victor Vaughan explained to Hewlett's successor Nellis Foster that the board of regents had granted funds to
equip a laboratory such as Hewlett envisioned, "but the money was
never expended because Doctor Hewlett decided to go to California."[47] Udo Wile, a dermatologist and syphilologist on the Michigan
faculty, shared Hewlett's frustration about laboratory facilities at the
hospital. He told the regents,

> the present laboratory, used by the students for routine ward
> work, has become too small for the present classes and moreover
> its location, immediately next to the Medical Amphitheatre, has
> made it impossible for my students to use the laboratory without
> disturbing those conducting lectures in the Amphitheatre.[48]

At this time, the hospital facilities at Michigan were also deemed
inadequate. Walter Sawyer informed Christian Holmes of Cincinnati
that the regents had approved the construction of a new hospital
because the existing facility was "out of date and inadequate."[49] New
clinical and laboratory facilities were planned, but Hewlett left the
University of Michigan before they were constructed. Although he
served with Victor Vaughan on the hospital committee of the medical
faculty, Hewlett and his fellow committee members had limited ability
to institute changes—finances were tightly controlled by the regents.[50]

---

46. H. Bishop Canfield to H. B. Hutchins, October 14, 1915, in Faculty Meeting
Minutes, 1914–17, University of Michigan Medical School Collection, Bentley Library.

47. Vaughan to Foster, March 25, 1916, in University of Michigan Medical School
Collection, miscellaneous correspondence, box 32, July 1916, A–N, Bentley Library.

48. Board of Regents, December 1, 1915, exhibit file, University of Michigan
Medical School Collection, Bentley Library.

49. Sawyer to Holmes, June 26, 1915, Walter Sawyer correspondence, June 1915
folder, Bentley Library.

50. Peterson and Shaw, "University Hospital," 970–71.

According to Frank Wilson, when Hewlett's successor Nellis Foster arrived in Ann Arbor in 1916, he

> found the [internal medicine] department established in the old Medical Ward.... This building had twenty-three beds, and there was no formal outpatient service. A small room, measuring about five by ten feet, provided the only available space for experimental work.[51]

Vaughan realized the implications of such modest facilities. Although he was proud that Michigan had "furnished its quota of scientific medical men to the ranks of the profession in this country," he informed the university's president that the integrity of his faculty was threatened:

> It is true that greater financial reward and especially more abundant provision for research work have from time to time taken from us some of our best men. This will continue from time to time. As I now write these lines, another university medical school is contemplating offering one of our best men a larger salary and possibly greater opportunity for productive research.[52]

Vaughan shared Hewlett's belief that adequate laboratory facilities were critical for the practice of modern medicine as well as for the pursuit of research. He informed a physician in Colorado in 1916,

> No hospital can be considered as properly equipped which is not supplied with complete laboratory facilities. The diagnosis of disease depends now largely upon laboratory tests. The hospital must have in it, or at its service, chemical, pathological, serological, and X-Ray laboratories.

---

51. Wilson, "Department of Internal Medicine," in Shaw, *University of Michigan*, 2: 841.

52. Vaughan to Harry B. Hutchins, "Report from the Dean of the Medical School," [September 1915], University of Michigan Medical School Collection, box 32, September 1915, Bentley Library.

Vaughan felt larger institutions should equip their laboratories for research as well as for routine clinical tests.[53]

Hewlett and Vaughan knew what would attract high-quality physicians to Ann Arbor—modern and well-equipped facilities, capable colleagues, and a dedicated staff. But the success of the medical school and its hospital also depended on patients coming to Ann Arbor for evaluation and treatment. Students and interns actively participated in the care of patients at University Hospital, and the quality of this care was of concern to Hewlett when he arrived in Ann Arbor. Although he was an advocate of active involvement of medical students in the wards, he was troubled by the amount of responsibility given them at Michigan.

He informed the university's executive secretary:

> There are at present in the hospital two classes of Internes. The first are doctors and the second students. When I came to Ann Arbor I found students acting as Medical Internes. I am personally very much opposed to this practice, because the Interne has the entire control of the patients in the absence of the visiting staff. With a continual succession of students acting in this capacity, I feel that the hospital is in danger of some very unpleasant situations, possibly even of law suits.

Hewlett asked that two of his assistants be permitted to serve as his interns during the coming year.[54]

The hospital was having difficulty recruiting interns when Hewlett arrived. Reuben Peterson, the medical director, went so far as to describe those who were on the staff as "inferior men." In a 1915 memorandum to university president Harry Hutchins, Peterson attributed this to the lack of suitable housing for the interns prior to 1911. Before then, he wrote, "the hospital was in the humiliating position of seeing her best senior students applying for intern positions elsewhere."

---

53. Vaughan to R. W. Corwin, April 24, 1918, University of Michigan Medical School Collection, miscellaneous correspondence, box 32, July 1916, A–N, Bentley Library.

54. Hewlett to Shirley Smith, December 16, 1908, attached to Smith to Walter Sawyer, December 19, 1908, in Walter Sawyer Correspondence, December 1908 file, Bentley Library.

He explained,

> While the young physician will cheerfully sacrifice much for the sake of practical hospital experience, he drew the line at the quarters and food offered him by our hospital. The best men went elsewhere for their experience. We had to be satisfied with inferior men, who were continually getting the hospital into trouble by their ignorance and lack of tact.

Peterson informed Hutchins, "All this has been changed by the interns' home where the men are comfortably housed and provided." The quality of the interns had improved, and Peterson boasted, "the different departments of the hospital have so arranged their intern services that the experience offered to the young physician is among the best in the country."[55] Hewlett could take some of the credit for improving the postgraduate training program in medicine at Michigan.

Even if the facilities were inadequate, the financial situation at University Hospital was improving during the last year of Hewlett's tenure in Ann Arbor. In just one year, profits had improved dramatically, patient days had increased, and the total number of patients registered had grown as well.[56]

So, things were going well in 1916 at the University of Michigan medical school and at its hospital. They were also going well for Hewlett. His monograph *Functional Pathology of Internal Diseases* had been published and was receiving excellent reviews. Pathologic physiology, which Hewlett had done so much to popularize in America, was gaining recognition. Thomas Boggs of Johns Hopkins, another of Krehl's pupils, claimed in 1916, "The importance of physiological thinking and the recognition of disturbed function as the basis of symptomatology are hard to overemphasize: and the American teachers and students are recognizing these facts more broadly each year."[57]

---

55. Peterson to Hutchins, August 9, 1915, "Reports of the Medical School," Harry Hutchins Papers, box 20, Bentley Library.

56. From Shirley Smith to Walter Sawyer, December 17, 1915, Walter Sawyer correspondence, December 1915 folder, Bentley Library.

57. Thomas Boggs, "Review of the Basis of Symptoms, the Principles of Clinical Pathology, by Dr. Rudolph [sic] Krehl," *Johns Hopkins Hosp. Bull.* 27 (1916): 367.

In 1916, Ray Wilbur, whom Hewlett knew from his days at Cooper Medical College, was elected president of Stanford University. Wilbur was professor of medicine and dean of the medical faculty at Stanford Medical School in San Francisco when he was chosen as the parent institution's president. He had attempted to woo Hewlett back to California as early as 1911, less than three years after he arrived in Ann Arbor. Then he asked Hewlett, "Is there any possibility that you yourself would consider a professorship in Medicine here with charge of the work at the City & County Hospital?"[58] If the description of this hospital by Stanford physician and historian Gunther Nagel is accurate, it is not surprising Hewlett turned down Wilbur's offer. Nagel claimed, "the old City and County Hospital was a two-story frame building with long corridors. It harbored far more rats than patients."[59]

Although this opportunity was not sufficient to draw Hewlett away from the University of Michigan, Wilbur kept trying. In 1914, he informed Hewlett, "We are still anticipating your coming out next summer and taking up some of your work here in our building. If you can give me an idea of what you want we will try to see if we can get it together for you."[60] Hewlett spent the summer of 1915 writing his monograph on pathologic physiology at the Lane Medical Library at Stanford's medical campus in San Francisco.

Later that year, Wilbur's chair at the Stanford Medical School was offered to Hewlett. This time Hewlett decided to return to his native California to join the institution that had taken over Cooper Medical College where his medical career had begun two decades earlier. Wilbur recalled,

> I was much pleased with Hewlett's appointment. I said at the time that "there is no better man of his age in clinical medicine in this country." He was a native Californian, had worked in the Stanford laboratories and on the faculty of the Cooper Medical

---

58. Wilbur to Hewlett, May 10, 1911, Stanford M553, box 1C, Albion Walter Hewlett folder, Lane Library.

59. Gunther W. Nagel, *A Stanford Heritage: Sketches of Ten Teacher-Physicians whose Standards of Excellence Became the Hallmark of a School of Medicine* (Stanford: Stanford Medical Alumni Association, 1970), 61.

60. Wilbur to Hewlett, April 8, 1914, Hewlett folder, Lane Library.

College before he went to Michigan, and was thoroughly familiar with conditions here on the Coast.[61]

In December 1915, Hewlett informed his colleagues at Michigan that he would leave Ann Arbor the following summer to become professor of medicine at Stanford.[62] Vaughan told Howard Agnew of the University of Alabama School of Medicine, "I greatly regret Dr. Hewlett's leaving us. It will be a task not altogether pleasant to find someone to fill his place."[63] During Hewlett's final faculty meeting at Michigan, Vaughan voiced his appreciation of Hewlett's contributions to the medical school and the university.[64] In assessing Hewlett's tenure at Michigan, Frank Wilson emphasized his productivity in clinical research and the beneficial effect this had on his associates. He characterized Hewlett as intellectually honest, unselfish, modest, and altruistic.[65] The Michigan faculty were aware of their loss.

Victor Vaughan was familiar with the new Stanford medical school. He had visited San Francisco and Palo Alto in 1914 to make a formal evaluation of its medical department and was impressed by what he saw. He informed Stanford's president that the laboratories were well appointed and well staffed, the faculty of the scientific branches was of excellent quality, the medical library was among the best in the country, the hospital—although somewhat out-of-date— was well managed, and the outpatient department was serving the patients well at the same time it provided an excellent learning experience for the students. Vaughan urged the Stanford officials to continue to support their new medical department and assured them that philanthropists would soon contribute to the institution if it continued its commitment to research.[66] Hewlett was, therefore, going to an institution whose heritage he knew and whose future appeared most promising.

---

61. Robinson and Edwards, *Ray Lyman Wilbur*, 208.

62. Faculty Meeting Minutes, December 10, 1915, University of Michigan Medical School Collection, Bentley Library.

63. Vaughan to Agnew, January 24, 1916, [copy] in University of Michigan Medical School Collection, miscellaneous correspondence, box 32, July 1916, A–L, Bentley Library.

64. Faculty Meeting Minutes, June 22, 1916, Bentley Library.

65. Wilson, "The Department of Internal Medicine."

66. Vaughan to J. C. Branner, June 9, 1914, Faculty Minutes, Stanford School of Medicine, box 1, Lane Library.

Personal considerations also contributed to Hewlett's decision
to leave Ann Arbor after only eight years. He was a native Californian
and had married Louise Redington in San Francisco just before moving to Ann Arbor in 1908. The couple had two children while they
lived in Ann Arbor, Louise in 1909 and William in 1913. The children's grandparents lived in the San Francisco area. Returning to
California would allow frequent family gatherings, which were impossible if Hewlett remained in Ann Arbor or accepted an offer from
an Eastern school.

Before his departure for California in the summer of 1916, Hewlett summarized his eight years at Michigan: "These years have witnessed an extraordinary growth in our University Hospital, a growth
which has established the proposition that in this country, as in Germany, a large university hospital can be developed in a small city."
His experience at Michigan proved to Hewlett that "patients are willing to travel considerable distances in order to receive expert medical
attention." He recounted the dramatic advances in medical diagnos-
tics—his own special interest—during his career. The increasingly
complex tests and growing demand for them led him to conclude,

> In order to render an efficient diagnostic service in the future it
> will be necessary either to increase the number of beds at the
> disposal of the department [of internal medicine] or to reorganize
> the out-patient service in such a manner that out-patients can
> be submitted to a fuller routine examination by a group of assis-
> tants.

In his address, Hewlett hinted at his frustration with the facilities
at his disposal in Ann Arbor. In Hewlett's opinion, a university had
a responsibility to support research, and the members of the medical
department of a university should actively participate in clinical investigation. But, if talented individuals were to "devote their best
years to the university side of medicine," they must be provided with
adequate facilities for research. Newer methods in biochemistry,
physiology, bacteriology, and immunology required sophisticated
apparatus, skilled assistants, and space.

Hewlett concluded,

> Herein it seems to me has been the most serious defect in my
> department. Our facilities for the study of cardiovascular disease

have been excellent but only beginnings have been made along other lines. The growth of the Hospital has been so rapid and the demand for more beds and for a larger staff of physicians and nurses so insistent that requests for larger and more efficient laboratories must often have seemed trivial. But we should remember that size is only one factor in the constitution of a great clinic.

Hewlett was a cautious supporter of the expansion of the full-time system from the scientific branches of medicine to the clinical disciplines. He explained, "It is becoming evident that if the members of the clinical staff are to do research in addition to their hospital and teaching duties, there will be relatively little time left for private practice." Nevertheless, he believed that students should be exposed to physicians in private practice to avoid the "disadvantage of bringing them in contact solely with men who devote themselves to the scientific side of medicine."[67] The University of Michigan had not adopted the strict full-time system for its clinical teachers. Victor Vaughan informed Hewlett's successor Nellis Foster,

> You will certainly want to do some private work. It will be perfectly proper for you as Professor of Medicine in this School to do consultation work. . . . I certainly hope that in time you will become a popular consultant, but not popular enough to interfere with your University duties.[68]

Hewlett had a vision for Michigan—a vision he would attempt to bring into existence at Stanford. He told his audience,

> The University Hospital has reached a size that is adequate or nearly adequate for its university purposes, and it seems to me that the time is at hand when more effort should be made toward its development as a center of clinical research. In the appointment of my successor a step in this direction has been made. Dr.

---

67. Albion Walter Hewlett, "Eight Years in the Department of Internal Medicine," *Trans. Clin. Soc. Univ. Mich.* 7 (1916): 146–49.

68. Vaughan to Foster, June 23, 1916, in University of Michigan Medical School Collection, miscellaneous correspondence, box 32, June 1916, A–M, Bentley Library.

Foster has made important contributions in applying the methods and data of biochemistry to the solution of clinical problems and he is to have a chemical laboratory connected with his service. It seems to me that further encouragement to this and to similar lines of development must be given, if Michigan is to keep pace with the leaders in clinical medicine.[69]

Walter Hewlett and his wife put their children on a train for San Francisco in July 1916, and set out for California in their Overland motorcar on the so-called "Yellow Trail" that would take them through the northern states to California. They camped in farmers' fields, confronted hordes of mosquitos, were saturated by thunderstorms in their open car, and dealt with a variety of mechanical problems as their machine challenged America's primitive roads. They arrived at Hewlett's father's ranch in California at 11:00 at night a month after they left Ann Arbor.[70]

When Hewlett arrived in California, the Stanford Hospital was being constructed adjacent to the old Lane Hospital in San Francisco. When the new facility opened in December 1917, with accommodations for 125 private patients, the Lane Hospital became a teaching hospital. Shortly after Hewlett's return to San Francisco, his career was disrupted by World War I. He served as a lieutenant commander in the medical corps of the Naval Reserve and went abroad with the Stanford Base Hospital Unit, which was stationed at Strathpeffer, near Inverness, Scotland. Hewlett also served in France where he witnessed the great influenza pandemic, an experience that led him to write a valuable paper on the subject.

Life in America gradually returned to normal as the war came to a close. Hewlett remained committed to his agenda of encouraging

---

69. Hewlett, "Eight Years." See also Victor Vaughan, "The Medical School during the Administration of President Hutchins from October 1909 to June 1920," in Harry Hutchins file, University of Michigan Medical School Collection, miscellaneous correspondence, box 33, Bentley Library. Correspondence between Victor Vaughan and Nellis Foster, Hewlett's successor, provides a picture of the Department of Internal Medicine and clinical laboratory work at the University of Michigan at the time of Hewlett's departure. See especially Foster to Vaughan, March 20, 1916, in University of Michigan Medical School Collection, miscellaneous correspondence, box 32, July 1916, A–N, Bentley Library.

70. "The Diary of Louise Redington Hewlett: 'Following the Yellow Trail' from Ann Arbor, Michigan 7/2/16 to San Francisco, California 8/4/1916," kindly supplied by William Hewlett, Palo Alto.

the physiological approach to the diagnosis of disease—and to his belief that more adequate laboratory facilities were crucial for the practice of modern medicine and for the development of clinical research in America. In a 1919 report, he charged that the clinical laboratories at Stanford were not meeting the demands of the clinicians. Although simple examinations of blood and urine were satisfactory, some chemical or serological tests were "difficult or impossible to obtain." The Wassermann reaction, for example, was performed only twice a week "which sometimes causes irritating delays." Hewlett warned, "To attract progressive physicians Stanford Hospital should have available in its clinical laboratory the latest methods which may be of value in diagnosis or treatment." He urged a "radical change" in the organization of the laboratory: it should be more closely affiliated with the hospital and should be under the charge of a "clinical pathologist" whose main interest was diagnostic laboratory tests.[71]

Hewlett continued his investigations of cardiac arrhythmias and conduction disturbances at Stanford. He was one of the first to study the value of quinidine in atrial fibrillation. In addition, he undertook a series of investigations into the pathophysiology of dyspnea and continued his tradition of active teaching on the medical wards. Reflecting the era as much as the personality of the man, an air of formality characterized Hewlett's rounds at Stanford Hospital. Before he arrived on the ward at 7:30 A.M., the patients were bathed, their linen was changed, and bedpans and basins were placed out of sight. His head nurse recalled that Hewlett was reserved and gentlemanly: "A respectful decorum was maintained between the professor, the students, interns, and nurses which was never overstepped."[72]

Active in professional and scientific societies throughout his career, Hewlett served as president of the California Academy of Medicine in 1922. Three years later, he was elected president of the American Society for the Advancement of Clinical Investigation. He became ill during the summer of 1925 and died of a malignant brain tumor on November 14 of that year, at the age of fifty. His premature death took from America a pioneer of clinical investigation who cata-

---

71. [Albion Walter Hewlett], "Report of the Committee on the Clinical Laboratory," in "Minutes of the Clinical Committee of Stanford University," box 9, binder 4, p. 10, Lane Library.

72. Nagel, *Stanford Heritage*, 41–47.

lyzed the shift from pathological to physiological thinking among the nation's medical teachers and practitioners.

Stanford's president, Ray Wilbur, characterized Hewlett as

> a trained physiologist who developed into a skilled practitioner. . . . Throughout his life he was orderly, thorough, scientific and analytical and he became a brilliant teacher and man of medicine. . . . His heart was in the clinic and the laboratory. To bring them closer together was his ideal."[73]

J. Marion Read, an assistant in medicine at Stanford during most of Hewlett's tenure there, recalled Hewlett's intellectual honesty, his extensive fund of medical knowledge, and his humility. We also learn from Read that some perceived Hewlett as rather aloof, but he was, in Read's opinion, "delightfully human. He possessed a contagious laugh and thoroughly enjoyed a joke."[74] An avid outdoorsman, Hewlett enjoyed tennis and fishing and built a cabin at The Cedars, an enclave in the Sierra Nevada mountains popular with Stanford faculty members.

The year after Hewlett died, sixteen Stanford graduates established the Hewlett Club. This organization, which is still in existence, was a combination journal club and forum for the discussion and criticism of research being undertaken by its members.[75] At the first-anniversary meeting, one of the club's members recalled, "Although he was best known to physicians in general as a scientific worker, those of us who were privileged to have him for a teacher appreciated him more as a clinician . . . . Truly he was a rare combination of investigator, clinician and man."[76]

73. Ray Lyman Wilbur, "Appreciation," in Albion Walter Hewlett, *Pathological Physiology of Internal Diseases, Functional Pathology* (New York: D. Appleton & Co., 1928).

74. J. Marion Read, *A History of the California Academy of Medicine, 1870 to 1930* (San Francisco: California Academy of Medicine, 1930), 143–48.

75. "The Hewlett Club: Minutes of the meetings, 1926–1934," Lane Library.

76. Quoted in Harvey, "Albion Walter Hewlett," 212–13.

Cyrus Cressey Sturgis and American Internal Medicine, 1913–1957

Steven C. Martin

The career of Cyrus Sturgis spanned an extraordinary period in the history of American medicine. Between his enrollment at the Johns Hopkins University School of Medicine in 1913 and his retirement from the chairmanship of the University of Michigan's Department of Internal Medicine in 1957, intellectual and social forces revolution-ized the practice of medicine (fig. 7). Medical knowledge exploded, adding corticosteroids, cancer chemotherapy, penicillin and a host of diagnostic assays to the medical armamentarium. Once-peripheral subjects, such as genetics, and entirely new fields, such as nuclear medicine, developed into fundamental disciplines. Medical training expanded from medical school to include internship, residency, and fellowships. Physicians basked in the glow of unprecedented social prestige. The federal government emerged as the leading supporter of research, and research moved ever further away from the bedside and into the laboratory.[1] These dramatic developments during the

I would like to thank Joel Howell for his support, advice, and encouragement, the Department of Internal Medicine for the invitation to prepare this work, the many people I interviewed, and the librarians and staff at the Michigan Historical Collections, Countway Library, New York Academy of Medicine, Johns Hopkins University, and Albert Einstein College of Medicine. I would especially like to thank the Sturgis family for sharing their family scrapbook, their recollections, and their encouragement.

1. There is an enormous literature on the history of twentieth-century American medicine. Two useful sources that include information on the entire span of American medical history are: Rosemary Stevens, *American Medicine and the Public Interest* (New Haven: Yale University Press, 1971) and Paul Starr, *The Social Transformation of American Medicine* (New York: Basic Books, 1982). For the perspective of physicians who experienced these changes, see the special issue of *Daedalus* 14, no. 2 (Spring 1986), entitled "America's Doctors, Medical Science, Medical Care."

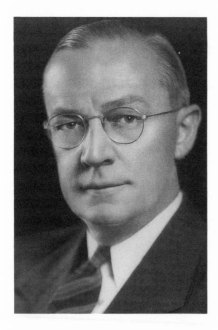

Fig. 7. Cyrus Cressey Sturgis

early and middle decades of this century reverberated throughout American medicine, leading many to label this period the "Golden Age of American Medicine."[2]

Yet nostalgia for this era and for its extraordinary accomplishments obscures the challenges faced by Sturgis and his colleagues. Change within medicine occurred in a volatile social environment. The impact of world events like the Depression, World War II, and the Korean conflict demanded creative responses. Even changes hailed as unequivocal medical advances created problems. A growing emphasis on specialization and an increasing reliance upon technology troubled many who feared these developments contained within them the seeds of a disquieting shift away from medicine's traditional emphasis on the care, as well as cure, of the patient. Within academia, departmental chairs wrestled with the appropriate division of resources between patient care, teaching, and research.

---

2. See John Burnham, "American Medicine's Golden Age: What Happened to It?" in Judith Walzer Leavitt and Ronald L. Numbers, eds., *Sickness and Health in America* (Madison: University of Wisconsin Press, 1985), 248–58.

As chairman of the Department of Internal Medicine from 1928 to 1957, Cyrus Sturgis grappled with all of these concerns. His story serves as an important case study of the issues facing internal medicine during the Golden Age, highlighting the difficult decisions American medicine faced and the options available as internal medicine developed into the discipline we recognize today.[3]

The Ambiguous World of Clinical Research: Cyrus Sturgis at Johns Hopkins Medical School

Sturgis was born in 1891 in Pendleton, Oregon. The son of a prominent banker, he attended Pendleton High School before pursuing premedical studies at the University of Washington. After graduating in 1913, he married his sweetheart Una Smith and headed east to Baltimore, matriculating to the Johns Hopkins University School of Medicine.[4]

Hopkins in this era was arguably the finest medical school in the United States, perhaps the world. Founded in 1893, it rapidly became the model for American medical schools, requiring a college degree for admission and adopting a four-year curriculum, with two years of basic sciences emphasizing laboratory work followed by two years of clinical instruction. Although Michigan stood at the forefront in agitating for many of these educational reforms,[5] it was at Hopkins that the entire model was first completely instituted.[6]

The philosophy with which Hopkins inculcated its students emphasized that science was the cornerstone of good medicine. How-

---

3. On the history of internal medicine, see Russell C. Maulitz and Diana E. Long, eds., *Grand Rounds: One Hundred Years of Internal Medicine* (Philadelphia: University of Pennsylvania Press, 1988).

4. Obituaries for Sturgis that include basic biographical information were published in the *Journal of the American Medical Association* 196, no. 12 (1966): 39 and the *University of Michigan Medical Bulletin* 32, no. 4 (1966): 207. See also *Annals of Internal Medicine* 41 (1954): 183 for biographical information.

5. See the chapter in this volume by Kenneth Ludmerer, "The University of Michigan Medical School: A Tradition of Leadership."

6. The history of Hopkins has been extensively documented. The most recent summary is its centennial history by A. McGehee Harvey, Gert H. Brieger, Susan L. Abrams, and Victor A. McCusick, *A Model of Its Kind* (Baltimore: Johns Hopkins University Press, 1989). On its impact on American medical education, see Kenneth M. Ludmerer, *Learning to Heal: The Development of American Medical Education* (New York: Basic Books, 1985).

ever, the definition of what constituted science, especially clinical science, remained ambiguous.[7] Two distinctly different approaches vied for supremacy during the years Sturgis attended Hopkins. Experimental physiology provided the first model. Sturgis was deeply influenced by Lewellys Barker, professor of medicine at Johns Hopkins, and a staunch advocate of experimental physiology.[8] For Barker, as for many influential young academics (including Michigan's Albion Walter Hewlett), experimental physiology represented a new and exciting approach to clinical problems. These men felt increasingly limited by the structural emphasis of anatomy and pathology and turned to physiology to help unravel the relationships between structure, function, and disease. The experimental physiologists argued that symptoms and disease represented more than structural abnormalities; they reflected deranged function, that is, disordered physiology.[9]

Physiology required a new approach to the acquisition of medical knowledge. Barker argued,

> What we need above all at this time are physicians and surgeons trained in physiology and pathology who will spend a part of their time in careful observation in the wards and over the operating table; who will there collect facts which will give them ideas

---

7. The meaning of science in medicine has received considerable attention from historians of medicine in recent years. The incisive essay by John Harley Warner, "Science in Medicine" in Sally Gregory Kohlstedt and Margaret W. Rossiter, eds., *Historical Writing on American Science* (Baltimore: Johns Hopkins University Press, 1985), 37–58, provides a superb overview that emphasizes the multiple meanings afforded to science in medicine.

8. Sturgis wrote Barker late in Barker's career that he remembered every detail of Barker's presentations in medical clinic. Sturgis to Barker, November 5, 1940, Sturgis file, Alan Mason Chesney Medical Archives, Johns Hopkins Medical Institutions, Baltimore, Md.

9. See Bruce Fye, *The Development of American Physiology* (Baltimore: Johns Hopkins University Press, 1987), especially 220–22 on Barker, and Gerald Geison, ed., *Physiology in the American Context, 1850–1940* (Bethesda, Md.: American Physiological Society, 1987). On Barker, see A. McGehee Harvey, Victor A. McKusick, and John D. Stobo, *Osler's Legacy: The Department of Medicine at Johns Hopkins, 1889–1989* (Baltimore: Department of Medicine, Johns Hopkins University, 1990), 19–25. In the Michigan context, see the chapter in this volume by W. Bruce Fye, "Albion Walter Hewlett: Teacher, Clinician, Scientist, and Missionary for Pathologic Physiology," whose wording I paraphrase when discussing the approach of experimental physiologists to symptoms.

to be submitted to experimental test, and who, during the rest of their time, will go down into the laboratories adjacent to the wards and actually make these experiments.[10]

For experimental physiologists, the questions might be derived from the wards, but the laboratory held the key to answering the questions.

The alternative, traditional approach to clinical research Sturgis experienced at Johns Hopkins was clinical observation. Classically, physicians had added to the corpus of medical knowledge by applying their observational skills at the bedside to derive important medical insights. In America, the man who epitomized this tradition was Sir William Osler, the first professor of medicine at Hopkins. Although Osler left Hopkins eight years before Sturgis arrived, his legacy was enormously powerful, and one can unhesitatingly assert that his philosophy directly influenced Sturgis.[11]

The science practiced by Osler was distinctly different from that practiced in the physiology lab. Osler described the task of clinical research:

To wrest from nature the secrets which have perplexed philosophers in all ages, to track to their sources the causes of disease, to correlate the vast stores of knowledge, that they may be quickly available for the prevention and cure of disease—these are our ambitions. To carefully observe the phenomena of life in all its phases normal and perverted, to make perfect the most difficult of all the arts, the art of observation, to call to aid the science of experimentation, to cultivate the reasoning faculty, so as to be able to know the true from the false.[12]

---

10. Lewellys F. Barker, "Medicine and the Universities," *American Medicine* 4 (1902): 146, quoted in Fye, *The Development of American Physiology*, 221.

11. Harvey, McKusick, and Stobo, *Osler's Legacy*, 1–18.

12. A. McGehee Harvey, *Science at the Bedside: Clinical Research in American Medicine, 1905–1945* (Baltimore: Johns Hopkins University Press, 1981), epigraph. It is interesting to note that Harvey chooses this quotation for the epigraph, highlighting not only the reverence for Osler that persists among academic physicians, but subtly implying that the observational science of Osler has never lost its importance to clinical research.

Osler gave primacy to clinical observation, with experimentation assuming a secondary role. It is not that Osler felt experimental science unimportant, but that its importance paled in comparison to clinical study *at the bedside*. Both Barker and Osler accepted observational and experimental methodologies as vitally important and mutually reinforcing, yet they chose distinctly different emphases.[13]

This struggle to define the nature of clinical research and to decide the relative importance of observation and experimentation is an important theme in the history of internal medicine during this era. At stake was more than an approach to research, for each methodologic approach also contained an implicit hierarchy of priorities for research, education, and patient care. The "observationalist" embraced teaching and clinical skills as essential to his or her task because they provided the environment and tools necessary for meticulous scientific observation. His or her science was anchored firmly to the bedside, where all three tasks were performed. In contrast, the experimentalist began at the bedside but turned away to the laboratory to discern the truth. (By the last quarter of the twentieth century, the experimentalist rarely appeared at the bedside.) The laboratory occupied the heights of the experimentalist hierarchy, with patient care and instruction necessarily subordinate. Although the comments of Barker and Osler describe an idealized harmony between observational and experimental approaches, it was a harmony that became increasingly difficult to realize as the century progressed.[14]

The tension between observational and experimental methodologies also carried implicit assumptions about who was qualified to pursue research. Observational techniques were presumably the property of all skilled physicians, but experimental techniques re-

---

13. Ludmerer comments on the generational difference between Osler and Barker and discusses the importance of Osler's willingness to accept laboratory science as a crucial element in the widespread acceptance of experimental science in *Learning to Heal*, 133–36. Although this is undoubtedly true, his comments underestimate the persistence of differences among academic physicians over the proper relationship between the laboratory and the bedside.

14. Two excellent essays, Gerald L. Geison, "Divided We Stand: Physiologists and Clinicians in the American Context," and Russell Maulitz " 'Physician versus Bacteriologist': The Ideology of Science in Clinical Medicine," in Charles Rosenberg and Morris Vogel, eds., *The Therapeutic Revolution* (Philadelphia: University of Pennsylvania Press, 1979), comment upon the tensions between clinicians and the emerging laboratory scientists. The tension within academic medicine, albeit less pronounced than that between practitioner and professor, has been underestimated.

quired specialized training. The conflict over scientific method implied different visions of the qualifications needed to succeed in academia. As research became increasingly associated with an experimentalist paradigm, departments of internal medicine became populated by full-time academicians whose research interests defined their professional identity. Professionalization based upon the experimentalist paradigm drove a wedge between practitioners and academics that did not exist for Osler.[15]

The maelstrom over defining the nature of academic internal medicine—who would occupy its professional ranks, what scientific methodology should be pursued, how its practitioners should balance patient care, teaching, and research—continued throughout Sturgis's career. The framework for ensuing debates was already discernible as Sturgis received his medical training. At Hopkins, the traditional approach of Osler remained deeply embedded in the local culture, but it rested cheek by jowl with the experimental approach that was gradually gaining ascendancy. Sturgis, throughout his career, struggled to achieve the harmonious ideal envisioned by both Barker and Osler. As the years passed, reconciling the experimental and observational approaches became more and more difficult.

Climbing the Academic Ladder: Sturgis at the Brigham

Sturgis performed extremely well at Hopkins and was elected a member of Phi Beta Kappa during his senior year.[16] When he sought an

---

15. The professionalization of academic medicine as a career path was a central element in the reform of American medical education. See Ludmerer, *Learning to Heal,* especially chapter 2. See also Donald Fleming, *William H. Welch and the Rise of Modern Medicine* (Baltimore: Johns Hopkins University Press, 1954, 1987) for the biography of a key figure in this process. This initial movement proved most successful in establishing full-time academic careers for medical school faculty in the basic sciences.

The process of professionalizing within academia was hardly unique to medicine during this era, and an interesting parallel phenomenon occurred within the biologic sciences. During the two decades surrounding the turn of the century, experimental biology began to dominate academic biology. See "Special Section on American Morphology at the Turn of the Century," *Journal of the History of Biology* 14 (1981): 83–191.

In both academic medicine and biology, the heirs to the traditional, nineteenth-century scientific approach—natural history in biology and clinical observation in medicine—were driven to the fringes of academia. Both, however, remained legitimate elements within academic departments, especially in medicine. The clinical faculty did not become completely dominated by experimental scientists who professionalized as scientists.

16. French to Sturgis, March 10, 1917, Sturgis family scrapbook.

internship following his graduation, he received a sterling letter of recommendation from Theodore Janeway, physician-in-chief of the Johns Hopkins Hospital:

> Mr. C. C. Sturgis, a member of our graduating class, has done extremely good work in all subjects throughout his course, and his work in Medicine has been of exceptional excellence. It gives me great pleasure to recommend him as a man of solid attainments, a gentleman and a most desirable member for the staff of any hospital. Only the fact that he is married stands in the way of his receiving appointment in our hospital.[17]

In an era when physicians were expected to exhibit priestly devotion to their profession, the Hopkins proviso against married house staff was common, and forced Sturgis to seek a residency elsewhere. Janeway's comment that Sturgis was a gentleman is also noteworthy. Having the proper background, bearing, and behavior was essential to advancing up medicine's career ladder. Janeway's stamp of approval was more than polite social commentary; it was a critically important qualification.

With such a strong recommendation, Sturgis had little difficulty in securing one of the coveted internships offered by the Department of Medicine at Boston's Peter Bent Brigham Hospital. The Brigham, closely affiliated with Harvard Medical School, was another of American medicine's elite institutions. It was home to an extraordinary collection of physicians, led by its physician-in-chief, Henry A. Christian, and its surgeon-in-chief, Harvey Cushing. The connections established at the Brigham, especially with Henry Christian, would fundamentally shape the remainder of Sturgis's career.

America's entry into World War I coincided with the completion of Sturgis's internship, and Sturgis joined the U.S. Army Medical Corps. Through Christian's intervention,[18] he was assigned to U.S. Army General Hospital No. 9 in Lakewood, New Jersey, a Harvard-

---

17. Janeway to "Whom it may concern," December 12, 1916, Sturgis family scrapbook.

18. Sturgis to Christian, September 2, 1918, Henry A. Christian Papers, Francis A. Countway Library of Medicine, Harvard Medical School, Boston.

staffed hospital. At Lakewood, under the supervision of Francis W. Peabody, Sturgis began his career as an investigator.

Sturgis and Peabody focused their investigations on "soldier's heart." This syndrome consisted of a vague constellation of symptoms that were difficult to interpret or manage. Hundreds of soldiers in apparently good health, without evidence of organic heart disease, complained of fatigue, nervousness, irritability, chest pain, shortness of breath, and palpitations. The Army Medical Corps desperately struggled to understand the etiology, prognosis, and management of this syndrome, because it robbed the army of active personnel and because it proved uncomfortably difficult to distinguish from malingering.[19]

Peabody and Sturgis began their investigations by focusing on two physiologic conditions that induced many of the symptoms of soldier's heart: stimulation of the sympathetic nervous system and hyperthyroidism. Sturgis's first paper, entitled "Epinephrine and Soldier's Heart," examined the response of patients and controls to injections of epinephrine, in the belief that differential sensitivity to adrenalin and related compounds might explain the syndrome. His next paper, "Effects of the Injection of Atropine on the Pulse Rate, Blood Pressure and Basal Metabolism in Cases of Effort Syndrome," similarly pursued the issue of the function of the autonomic nervous system in soldier's heart.[20] Both papers demonstrate Sturgis and Peabody's adoption of the new paradigm of experimental physiology in clinical research.

Yet Sturgis also pursued a series of studies of soldier's heart that employed a traditional observational approach to clinical research. In these studies, no experimental intervention was performed; instead the investigator simply compiled data on readily observable phenomena.[21] Sturgis's research highlights how readily investigators

19. Joel D. Howell, "'Soldier's Heart': The Redefinition of Heart Disease and Specialty Formation in Early Twentieth Century Great Britain," *Medical History* supplement no. 5 (1985): 34–52.

20. Cyrus C. Sturgis, "Epinephrine and Soldier's Heart," *J.A.M.A.* 71 (1918):1912; Cyrus C. Sturgis, Joseph T. Wearn, and Edna N. Tompkins, "Effects of the Injection of Atropine on the Pulse Rate, Blood Pressure, and Basal Metabolism in Cases of 'Effort Syndrome'," *American Journal of Medical Science (Philadelphia)* 158 (1919):496–502.

21. Francis W. Peabody and Cyrus C. Sturgis, "Clinical Studies on the Respiration," *Archives of Internal Medicine* 29 (1922):277–305.

during this era incorporated both research styles, drifting easily between bedside and laboratory, each research approach accepted as independently important and the two seen as mutually reinforcing. For a brief time, the harmony envisioned by Osler and Barker remained undisturbed.

After the war, Sturgis returned to the Brigham and finished his residency. Upon its completion, he remained at the Brigham and garnered the prestigious position of assistant in the private practice of the hospital's physician-in-chief, Henry A. Christian. As a practitioner-investigator, Sturgis continued to pursue clinical research. But if, in the army, Sturgis had been influenced by Peabody, a strong advocate of experimental medicine,[22] his new mentor was Christian, whose philosophy was more in the Oslerian tradition. Gradually Sturgis's studies became more observational and less experimental.[23]

As Sturgis gained prominence at Harvard, he climbed the academic ladder. He presented at important scientific meetings sponsored by the Interurban Clinical Club and the New York Academy of Medicine. He was elected to membership in prestigious organizations and was promoted from teaching fellow through instructor to assistant professor at the Harvard Medical School.

Sturgis's emergence as a rising star in the Harvard system soon brought job offers from rival academic centers. As early as 1922, shortly before the completion of his residency, Sturgis was contacted by the Mayo Clinic and offered a position.[24] Despite being offered the handsome salary of $6,000, which during negotiations was raised to $7,500 with a promise of annual increases of $1,000, Sturgis elected to stay in Boston, lured by the promise of working alongside Christian. (The financial offer by Christian was probably also substantial, for the salary promised by the Harvard Corporation was a mere $2,300).[25]

---

22. Peabody was the first director of Harvard's Thorndike Memorial Laboratory, a key institution for the training of experimental clinical researchers. See Maxwell Finland, ed., *The Harvard Medical Unit at Boston City Hospital* (Boston: Harvard Medical School, 1982).

23. See, for example, Cyrus C. Sturgis, "Observations on One Hundred and Ninety Two Consecutive Days of the Basal Metabolism, Food Intake, Pulse Rate, and Body Weight in a Patient with Exophthalmic Goiter," *Archives of Internal Medicine* 32 (1923):50–73.

24. Wilder to Sturgis, June 21, 1922, and July 27, 1922, Sturgis family scrapbook.

25. Endicott to Sturgis, October 1, 1922, Sturgis family scrapbook.

In 1925 the University of Texas recruited Sturgis to become chair of the department of medicine, with the dean noting that the university had substantial resources. His comments showed remarkable foresight, informing Sturgis that "the University has lately struck oil on University lands," and adding that "at the present time we are deriving $900,000 a year from royalties on oil." The Dean concluded, "I believe within 10 years the University of Texas will be one of the wealthiest institutions of learning in the land."[26] Despite the rosy economic forecast, a salary of $5,000, and permission to generate additional income via private practice, Sturgis elected to remain at Harvard.

It would require an exceptionally attractive offer to lure Sturgis away from the comfortable environs of Boston, an offer that would emerge from a concatenation of events occurring in Ann Arbor.

Setting the Scene: The Department of Medicine and the Creation of the Simpson Institute

In the 1920s, Michigan's Department of Internal Medicine was heir to a proud tradition of excellence. However, after Walter Albion Hewlett left in 1916, the department entered a chaotic period in its history. In the decade between Hewlett's departure and Sturgis's arrival, five different men occupied the chairman's post. At one point, the school was unable to attract a suitable candidate and the chairmanship was briefly held by a radiologist. It was clear by the middle 1920s that the department required reinvigoration.[27]

The catalyst for this reinvigoration was the creation of the Thomas Henry Simpson Institute for Medical Research. Simpson was a wealthy industrialist who had earned a fortune in the iron industry. Late in his life, he developed pernicious anemia, at the time a disease both mysterious and incurable. After his death, his family founded a research institute devoted to discovering a cure for pernicious ane-

---

26. Keillen(?) to Sturgis, March 17, 1925, Sturgis family scrapbook.

27. Frank N. Wilson, "The Department of Internal Medicine," in Wilfred Shaw, ed., *The University of Michigan: An Encyclopedic Survey*, 2 (Ann Arbor: University of Michigan Press, 1951), 833–42, and Horace W. Davenport, *Fifty Years of Medicine at The University of Michigan: 1891–1941* (Ann Arbor: University of Michigan Medical School, 1986), 275–90.

mia, donating over $400,000 to the University of Michigan in 1924 to create such a facility.[28]

The donation by the Simpson estate highlights several important themes that characterized medical research during the interwar period. Donations by private philanthropy represented the single most-important source of funding for medical research. The Rockefeller Foundation created the first major research institute in the United States with the opening of the Rockefeller Institute in 1910. The establishment of this institute created a model for clinical research that was widely copied. Privately funded independent research institutes, often associated with a university or medical school, began to be established. The Simpson Institute fit easily into the pattern typified by such institutions, as did the McCormack Institute at the University of Chicago and the Wistar Institute at the University of Pennsylvania.[29]

In these institutes devoted to clinical research, researchers were committed to bringing the laboratory and the bedside closer together. Their physical plants embodied this philosophy by placing investigators' research laboratories in close proximity to their patients or subjects. The Simpson Institute design provided for nine patients in the same building that housed the scientific laboratories.[30]

In addition to illustrating the importance of private funding and clinical research, the Simpson Institute reflected another important trend in the evolution of support for medical research: the donation of funds directed at specific diseases. As disease advocacy groups, ranging from the National Association for the Prevention of Blindness to the American Society for the Control of Cancer, gained prominence during the 1920s, it became common for benefactors to direct funds to specific problems.[31]

---

28. Cyrus C. Sturgis, "First Annual Report of the Director of the Thomas Henry Simpson Memorial Institute for Medical Research," in *The University of Michigan President's Annual Report, 1927–1928* (Ann Arbor: University of Michigan, 1928) and Chris Zarafonetis, "The Thomas Henry Simpson Memorial Institute for Medical Research: Fortieth Anniversary," in Chris Zarafonetis, ed., *Proceedings of the International Conference on Leukemia-Lymphoma* (Philadelphia: Lea and Febiger, 1968), 7–12.

29. Harvey, *Science at the Bedside*.

30. Sturgis, "The First Annual Report of the Thomas Henry Simpson Memorial Institute for Medical Research."

31. On the role of the National Society for the Prevention of Blindness, see Stevens, *American Medicine and the Public Interest*, 102, and Bert Hansen, "What Perpetu-

The creation of the Simpson Institute naturally led to a search for a director. The dean of the Medical School, Hugh Cabot, seized upon this opening not only to recruit a director for the institute but also to obtain a new chairman for the Department of Medicine. The Institute provided both the resources and the opportunity necessary to lure Sturgis from his comfortable Boston existence.

The Search for a Director

The choice of Sturgis as the new director was far from obvious. Although Sturgis was a well-established investigator by this time, virtually none of his research had anything to do with hematology. His only connection with hematology research had been to refer private patients to the research team of George Minot and William Murphy, who were investigating pernicious anemia.[32] Ironically, between the donation of the endowment and the initiation of a search for Simpson's first director, this research led to a treatment for pernicious anemia. In 1925, Minot and Murphy established that patients fed a diet enriched with huge amounts of liver could be cured of pernicious anemia, a finding that was rewarded with the Nobel Prize.[33]

When Michigan began to search for a director for Simpson, Dean Cabot, who had come to Michigan from Harvard, contacted George

---

ates a Preventable Disease? A Political History of Infant Blindness," paper delivered at the 1988 annual meeting of the American Association for the History of Medicine. See also James Patterson, *The Dread Disease: Cancer and Modern American Culture* (Cambridge: Harvard University Press, 1987). As an example of the modern incarnation of this process, see Patrick Fox, "From Senility to Alzheimer's Disease: The Rise of the Alzheimer's Disease Movement," *Milbank Quarterly* 67 (1989):58–102.

32. The only article relating to hematology that Sturgis published prior to reaching Michigan was Matthew Riddle and Cyrus Sturgis, "Basal Metabolism in Chronic Myelogenous Leukemia," *Archives of Internal Medicine* 39 (1927):255–74. The referral of the patient to Minot and Murphy is documented on the hospital chart reproduced in Lawrence Kass, *Pernicious Anemia* (Philadelphia: W. B. Saunders, 1976), 1–62.

33. George Minot and William P. Murphy, "Treatment of Pernicious Anemia by a Special Diet," *Journal of the American Medical Association* 87 (1926):470–76. See also Kass, *Pernicious Anemia*, 1–62, and the entries by Steven C. Martin in Daniel M. Fox, Marcia Meldrum, and Ira Rezak, eds., *Nobel Laureates in Physiology or Medicine* (New York: Garland Press, 1990).

Minot.[34] Minot's letter to Cabot provides a marvelous window into the criteria used during this era for the hiring of faculty for a major research and administrative position.

> Let me say personally, for the best interests of the University of Michigan, I fear Dr. [Raphael] Isaacs would not fill your position suitably. Not because of his inability or brilliance, but because of his birthright. He is the very best sort of a Jew and of the purest type. [Isaacs was an orthodox Jew.] This makes him a good individual laboratory worker, and he is most helpful, sympathetic, a perfect gentleman, but I am afraid he would never do to lead an investigative institution.

Lest it be implied that Minot was only concerned with the issue of Jews in academia, his comments about Murphy followed: "As for Murphy; his full name is William Parry Murphy; not an Irishman; excellent American; home Oregon," revealing that being Irish was also not considered a useful qualification for receiving an important academic position.[35]

This is not to assert that Minot himself was a bigot—in fact he maintained a warm relationship with Isaacs throughout his career[36]— but rather to emphasize that racism permeated American society during this era and medicine was hardly an exception. Just as Sturgis's appointment as an intern at the Brigham required Janeway's approval that he was a "gentleman," the criteria for advancement a decade later continued to include a complex mixture of personal, social, educational, and academic qualifications.

---

34. Minot is a central figure in the development of American hematology. As director of the Thorndike Memorial Laboratory, he emphasized the experimentalist approach and encouraged the growth of academic hematology along this model. His career is a useful contrast to Sturgis's experience at the Simpson Institute. See William Castle, "The Contributions of George Richards Minot to Experimental Medicine," *New England Journal of Medicine* 247 (1952): 585–91.

35. Minot to Cabot, May 25, 1926, University of Michigan Medical School (hereafter referred to as UMMS), dean's records, box 37, folder S1927, Bentley Historical Library, University of Michigan (hereafter, Bentley Library).

36. See Roger D. Isaacs, "Raphael Isaacs," unpublished manuscript, Francis A. Countway Library, Harvard Medical School, Boston, Mass. Minot was aware of the sensitivity of his comments, for he ends his remarks about Isaacs with the comment, "I should prefer you did not show this note to nobody [sic]." Minot to Cabot, May 25, 1926.

Dean Cabot's first choice was William Murphy. Despite initial interest, negotiations foundered when the search committee reached a consensus that "Dr. Murphy requires too great a salary and a budget." The early search for a candidate was not fruitful, including, apparently, a brief consideration of Sturgis in June of 1925. In October of that year, when Dean Cabot wrote to the Mayo Clinic requesting Will Mayo's assistance in finding a candidate, he noted that "We have searched the field pretty thoroughly without finding a satisfactory person."[37]

As construction neared completion in early 1926, the Simpson Institute remained leaderless. Mrs. Simpson began to exert pressure to find a director and made it clear that she would not approve of opening the Institute until a permanent director was recruited. Under this pressure, Cabot intensified his search and apparently reconsidered candidates he had previously rejected. Despite Minot's comments—and to the University of Michigan's credit—both Isaacs and Sturgis were contacted in November 1926.[38]

Under considerable pressure from Mrs. Simpson's edict, negotiations with Sturgis proceeded rapidly, and Cabot soon offered Sturgis not only the directorship of Simpson but also the chairmanship of the Department of Medicine. The offer of chairmanship was a secret agreement and provided that one year after arriving to take charge of Simpson, Sturgis would be appointed "Director of the Department of Medicine." Cabot cautioned that "We believe it very important that this arrangement in regard to taking over control [of Medicine] should not be discussed outside at the present time. This year would give you opportunity to make many decisions in regard to personnel, which should, I think, be made only after careful consideration on the ground." The offer included a salary of $15,000 and substantial research support.[39]

The need to move quickly to placate the Simpson family is highlighted by the speed with which the entire process occurred. Michi-

---

37. Search Committee to Cabot, and Cabot to Mayo, both in UMMS, dean's records, box 36, folder M1925.

38. Cabot to Little, November 11, 1926, UMMS, dean's records, box 37, folder S1927. See also Sturgis, "First Annual Report of the Simpson." Cabot to Isaacs, November 16, 1926, Cabot to Sturgis, November 24, 1926 and December 22, 1926, UMMS, dean's records, box 37, folder S1927.

39. Cabot to Sturgis, December 22, 1926, UMMS, dean's records, box 37, folder S1927.

gan contacted Sturgis on November 24, 1926, and he accepted the position on January 6, 1927. The board of regents accepted his appointment that evening, and President C. C. Little wired Sturgis the good news at 2:20 A.M.[40]

Sturgis Arrives in Ann Arbor

The appointment of Sturgis as the first director of Simpson and its formal dedication received extensive publicity in both the lay and medical press. Not only did the Boston and Detroit papers carry the announcement, but a wire service bulletin was issued. Leading medical publications, including *Science*, the *Journal of the American Medical Association*, and the *Boston Medical and Surgical Journal* also carried the announcement.[41]

The dedication ceremonies for the Thomas Henry Simpson Institute for Medical Research were held on February 10, 1927 (fig. 8). Sturgis, demonstrating the administrative and political savvy that would mark his career, invited his mentor Henry Christian to deliver the keynote address. Christian's address, which was reprinted in *Science*, admirably captures the atmosphere, promise and excitement of early twentieth century medical research.

> Through all the ages there has been some form of quest to fire the zeal of man. In the days of chivalry such a quest was typified by the search for the Holy Grail . . . . A little later and the quest took the form of exploration and settlement of new lands. Now, with unexplored lands almost non-existent, the quest has shifted to investigation, the search for truth and the discovery of new facts. Investigation has become the Holy Grail of science, and the quest in this form stirs the imagination and fires the zeal of a new type of Sir Galahad . . . . Pure, as typified by the search for the Holy Grail, is the purpose of this new institute for medical research.[42]

---

40. Sturgis to Little, January 6, 1927, and Little to Sturgis, January 7, 1927, Sturgis family scrapbook.

41. Clippings, n.d., Sturgis family scrapbook.

42. Henry A. Christian, "The Significance and Relationships of the Thomas Henry Simpson Memorial Institute for Medical Research," *Science* 65 (1927):359–61.

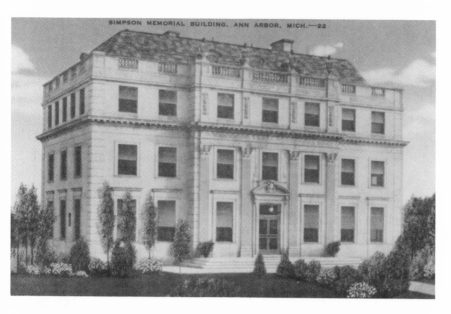

Fig. 8. The Simpson Institute. (From a postcard in the editor's collection.)

Even giving allowance for the rhetorical excess that typically accompanies dedicatory ceremonies, Christian touches here upon the extraordinary emotional appeal of medical research, not only—or even primarily—for its practitioners, but also for its patrons. It is often suggested that science and medicine developed into a kind of secular religion for Americans during the twentieth century, and it is precisely this impulse that one sees operating in Christian's comments.

Christian's address was filled with more than stirring rhetoric about the benefits of medical science. Christian, as an active clinician and a medical scientist of the older, Oslerian, observational school, worried about the potential conflict between clinical research and patient care. Christian declared that "patients guarantee . . . a research institute's being productive of good," but cautioned,

At the same time their presence places limitations on what may be done. The director is first of all responsible for the welfare of these patients. Nothing can be tried that is likely to injure them; nothing must be done without their free consent. In every hospital, and a clinical research institute is a hospital, the best possible care of the patients is the first duty of the institution, and all is secondary to this. In many experiments, desired combinations of conditions can be produced by the experimenter; with patients he must await the finding of the desired combination, as it has occurred independently of experiment. In this way clinical research may be infinitely slower than other forms of investigation.[43]

Once again, albeit in a slightly different configuration, tension emerges between a traditional medical approach, with its focus on the individual patient as the central concern of the physician, and the new scientific ethos that argued that the optimal care of individual patients would only result from the active, experimental pursuit of medical knowledge. The tension between patient care and clinical research has remained a central issue for clinical researchers.

Sturgis, like his mentor Christian, would devote considerable energy to trying to reconcile the needs of clinical research with the demands of patient care. Despite the growing trend in American medicine to emphasize research, Sturgis continued to embrace the sentiments Christian expressed in the dedicatory address, placing patient care at the center of his professional vision throughout his career.

Several challenges faced Sturgis when he arrived in Ann Arbor. He needed to stabilize the department of medicine after nearly a decade of turmoil. A research agenda for both the Simpson Institute and the rest of the department needed to be created. Teaching on the medicine services required immediate revision and the supervision of interns restructuring. Finally, he needed to establish a working relationship with the two full professors who antedated his arrival, Frank Wilson and L. H. Newburgh.

Sturgis and Pernicious Anemia

Sturgis's initial task at Michigan was to establish himself as an investigator of pernicious anemia. His first step in this direction was to

---

43. Ibid.

appoint Raphael Isaacs as assistant director of Simpson. Isaacs, who had worked closely with Minot, was a critical contributor to the early research performed at Simpson. Sturgis and Isaacs concentrated their initial efforts on improving the treatment of pernicious anemia. Although Minot and Murphy had discovered an effective form of therapy, it was a regimen that proved exceedingly difficult for patients to tolerate, requiring the daily ingestion of half a pound of broiled liver. Sturgis and colleagues sought to create a more efficient form of therapy, and in 1929 developed a preparation derived from hog stomachs that was one of the first, effective, parenteral treatments for pernicious anemia.[44]

A notable element in this discovery was the close collaboration between Sturgis and researchers at the Parke-Davis Company. When an effective product was created, the University and Parke-Davis reached a licensing arrangement that provided the University with royalties from the sale of the preparation, dubbed ventriculin, and required University approval of any use of the University's name in advertising for the product. The Simpson Institute provided quality control for the preparation by measuring the efficacy of individual lots of the product by using the only available assay for effectiveness—patient response. Sturgis's involvement with Parke-Davis illustrates the growing importance of interactions between academic medical scientists and the pharmaceutical industry, a relationship that provided the academics with critically needed funds for research and supplied their expertise, patient populations, and academic cachet to the pharmaceutical industry.[45]

The creation of ventriculin would be the last significant research Sturgis performed. As the years progressed, he became increasingly occupied by the administrative, service, and educational requirements of the chairmanship.

---

44. Cyrus Sturgis, "The Thomas Henry Simpson Memorial Institute for Medical Research," *President's Annual Report 1929–1930* (Ann Arbor: University of Michigan, 1930), 385–88. See also Cyrus C. Sturgis and Raphael Isaacs, "Use of Desiccated Hog Stomach in Pernicious Anemia," *Journal of the American Medical Association* 95 (1930):73.

45. Sturgis, *President's Annual Report 1929–1930*. On the relationship of academia and industry during this period, see John P. Swann, *Academic Scientists and the Pharmaceutical Industry: Cooperative Research in Twentieth-Century America* (Baltimore: Johns Hopkins University Press, 1988).

Sturgis as Administrator

In 1928, when Cyrus Sturgis assumed the chairmanship of the Department of Medicine, administering a department of internal medicine already presented a formidable challenge. The department contained six full faculty members, eight instructors, six research assistants, and eight interns. Its members contributed over twenty publications to the scientific literature that year. The department was responsible for the annual care of 2,700 inpatients and 23,000 outpatients at the recently opened University Hospital and provided instruction for over 300 junior and senior medical students.[46]

When Sturgis retired in 1957, he presided over a department of medicine that both quantitatively and qualitatively dwarfed its predecessor. The number of instructors in 1957 equaled the entire 1928 faculty. The faculty had more than doubled, now numbering fifty-six. The department had divided into specialty services, some of which had staffs that nearly equaled the size of the entire 1927 department. Admissions to the University Hospital's medicine services topped 4,000, and the medicine faculty were responsible for the instruction of nearly 800 medical students. The time, energy, and dollars committed to medical research had increased exponentially, and the faculty publications had increased sixfold.[47]

Historians have only recently begun to appreciate the significance of scientific administrators.[48] As the research enterprise grew ever more complex, effective scientific performance required a supportive bureaucratic infrastructure. The days of a scientist or physician working alone in a makeshift laboratory were disappearing rapidly as the twentieth century progressed and the requirements of space, equipment, and personnel—all of which ultimately translated

---

46. Data compiled from the *President's Annual Report 1928–1929* and *Medical School Announcement 1927–1928* (Ann Arbor: University of Michigan).

47. Data compiled from *President's Annual Report 1956–1957*, *Medical School Announcement 1956–1957*, and *Bibliography of Publications by Members of the Several Faculties of the University of Michigan, October 1, 1955 to September 30, 1957* (Ann Arbor: University of Michigan).

48. See, for example, Gerald Geison, *Michael Foster and the Cambridge School of Physiology* (Princeton: Princeton University Press, 1978), Robert Kohler, *From Medical Chemistry to Biochemistry* (New York: Cambridge University Press, 1982), and Robert E. Kohler, *Partners in Science: Foundations and Natural Scientists, 1900–1945* (Chicago: University of Chicago Press, 1991).

into money—became increasingly onerous. For investigators in an academic setting to become productive, they needed more than talent, they needed the resources and time that were controlled by scientific administrators.

The administrative responsibilities of academic internists like Sturgis decisively influenced more than the research enterprise. Because the department was responsible for patient care and teaching, these men had to balance conflicting demands and create priorities. Historians have primarily focused on the research production of academic departments and to date have failed to explore adequately the interrelationship of these issues within the context of academic medicine.

One brief example highlights these issues. Prior to Sturgis's arrival, the department was divided into separate services, including metabolism, cardiology, tuberculosis wards, and a private medical service. The service and teaching requirements of this arrangement demanded a substantial time commitment from the full-time faculty. Sturgis rearranged the department into four general medicine services. This administrative decision accomplished three goals: it reduced the service commitments of his premier researchers, Frank Wilson and L. H. Newburgh, it reformed medical training by providing senior faculty as attending physicians on all medicine services, and it implicitly challenged the trend toward specialization.[49]

During Sturgis's tenure, the issue of time for research versus service commitment remained a thorny problem. Sturgis's willingness to accommodate the needs of researchers is evident in his consistent support of Frank Wilson. Sturgis repeatedly excused Wilson from routine patient care and teaching. It is doubtful that Wilson would have functioned as a productive investigator without this kind of administrative support. Similarly, Sturgis acceded to Newburgh's request in 1938 to establish a specialized metabolism unit, despite his own preference for general medical services.[50]

Juggling conflicting demands and establishing priorities pro-

49. Wilson, *The University of Michigan: An Encyclopedic Survey*, 843.

50. Sturgis to Furstenberg, January 8, 1948, UMMS, dean's records, box 50, folder 1948S–T. "Memorandum in reference to the request of Dr. Newburgh to manage all diabetic patients on the medical services," September 28, 1938, cited in the chapter in this volume by Steven J. Peitzman, "Louis Harry Newburgh and Metabolism at Michigan."

vided the backdrop for Sturgis's decisions; the foreground was dominated by money. Financial problems revolved around two central themes: faculty salary and research support. Throughout his career, Sturgis battled the university for salary increases for his staff. He repeatedly warned that departmental morale and his ability to retain first-rate faculty were being undermined by the university's stingy reimbursement policy. Faculty were frequently wooed by competing universities promising higher salaries.[51]

Ironically, Sturgis's personal salary was quite handsome. In fact, after his hiring, Dean Cabot wrote to President Little to complain that the surgical faculty were grossly underpaid. Cabot noted that, in contrast to Sturgis's $15,000 salary, Cabot only received a salary of $5,000 plus a small income from private practice, while serving as a professor of surgery specializing in urology and as dean of the Medical School. Cabot remarked acerbically, "It might at least be suggested that if my work is satisfactory, I ought to receive more salary than a professor of medicine."[52]

Concern over faculty salaries for members of clinical departments had broader ramifications than faculty income and morale. The issue of faculty supplementing their salaries by maintaining private practices remained enormously divisive within the American medical establishment throughout Sturgis's tenure as chairman. On one side were the advocates of the so-called full-time plan, who argued that university faculty would have divided loyalties if they maintained private practices, and insisted that this arrangement be prohibited. The issue had been argued for the basic science faculty during the first two decades of the century, and by the 1920s, the vast majority of medical schools had adopted the full-time plan for their basic science faculty. In contrast, the advocates of full-time faculty status were unable to achieve the same consensus for the clinical faculty, and medical schools across the country developed a wide range of responses to the issue.[53]

Michigan's solution was to adopt a nominal full-time plan in

---

51. Sturgis to Wile, June 1, 1931, box 39, folder 1931–1932S and Sturgis to Furstenberg, November 29, 1949, box 51, folder Sm–Sz, UMMS, dean's records.

52. Cabot to Little, May 23, 1927, box 4, folder 13, C. C. Little Papers, Bentley Library.

53. See Ludmerer, *Learning to Heal,* and William Rothstein, *American Medical Schools and the Practice of Medicine* (New York: Oxford University Press, 1987).

1919. Although medical faculty were prohibited from private practice, surgeons' income was supplemented with clinical salaries. After the departure of Dean Cabot in 1930, when some departments became openly part-time, the Department of Medicine remained on the full-time plan.[54] In the late 1930s, Sturgis began to argue strenuously for the ability of some faculty to initiate part-time private practice, and Sturgis himself opened a small practice. Sturgis earnestly petitioned Dean Albert C. Furstenberg, who eventually succeeded Cabot and was Dean for the majority of Sturgis's tenure as chairman, to allow more members of his faculty to pursue practice. Sturgis argued that it was only through allowing the faculty to supplement their incomes in this way that the department could offer sufficient financial rewards to insure the retention of its faculty. The full-time controversy was never fully resolved during Sturgis's tenure.[55] The conflict between pure academic ideals and limited resources created a difficult situation that continues to haunt academic medical centers.

The financial support of research proved far less troublesome. One of Sturgis's greatest assets was his fund-raising ability. Throughout his career, Sturgis proved adept at securing funds from two key sources: private philanthropy and the pharmaceutical industry. The correspondence between Sturgis and Dean Furstenberg is replete with reports of support being garnered from such pharmaceutical firms as Parke-Davis, Upjohn, and Lilly.[56]

Private philanthropy was even more important, with members of the Department of Medicine soliciting funds from a host of different foundations. Sturgis once wrote Henry Christian that the Rackham Fund had set aside a million dollars as an endowment and added "I'm sure if more money were needed we could obtain it."[57] The success of similar efforts is highlighted by an exchange of letters between Sturgis and Furstenberg when Sturgis had grown tired of the bureaucracy required by a particular foundation and considered simply terminating the grant and applying elsewhere. Furstenberg

---

54. Davenport, *Fifty Years of Medicine*, 276–77, 314.

55. Sturgis to Furstenberg, June 29, 1940, April 11, 1945, and June 17, 1949, respectively, box 43, folder S, box 48, folder misc. S, and box 51, folder Sm–Sz, 1949, UMMS, dean's records.

56. See, for example, Sturgis to Furstenberg, July 15, 1937, and May 21, 1941, respectively, boxes 40 and 44, UMMS, dean's records.

57. Sturgis to Christian, October 2, 1937, Sturgis family scrapbook.

demurred, fearing such an action would foster the perception among foundations "that we [the University of Michigan] were inordinately wealthy with research funds."[58] Judging from the records, the foundations were probably right!

Another important characteristic of Sturgis's administrative style was humility. Sturgis remained comfortable within himself and did not demand that all power be centered in the chairman's office. For example, when the Rackham Foundation considered providing money for what was eventually to become the Rackham Arthritis Unit, Sturgis aggressively supported the proposal, writing the Rackham Foundation a detailed letter delineating the need for such research. Sturgis actively supported the Rackham grant despite the fact that it was explicitly designed to create a unit that was independent of the Department of Medicine. Similarly, when, after World War II, a Department of Genetics was established, Sturgis created no administrative roadblocks, despite the attitude of some that Genetics should remain subordinate to a clinical department.[59]

The humility of Sturgis's administrative style had disadvantages as well as advantages. In a department that contained strong personalities, Sturgis at times had difficulty controlling faculty members who were subordinate to him. Both Frank Wilson and L. H. Newburgh were not averse to going above Sturgis's head and requesting special privileges from either the dean or the university president. These episodes were a continuing source of annoyance and consternation to Sturgis. The attitude of Wilson and Newburgh may have stemmed in part from resentment of Sturgis. When Sturgis arrived from Harvard, where he had only achieved the rank of assistant professor, both Wilson and Newburgh were already full professors. Furthermore, each man developed a scientific stature significantly greater than Sturgis's and may well have bridled at their subordinate position. Their attitude must have smacked of ingratitude to Sturgis, for he often acceded to their requests for special treatment and vigorously supported their efforts to obtain funding and personnel.[60]

---

58. Furstenberg to Sturgis, May 18, 1945, box 48, UMMS, dean's records.

59. Sturgis to Horton, April 12, 1937, and Sturgis to Furstenberg, May 12, 1942, respectively, in boxes 41 and 45, UMMS, dean's records and personal communication, James Neel.

60. Sturgis to Furstenberg, November 16, 1943, and January 8, 1948, respectively, box 46, folder 1943S, and box 50, folder S–T, UMMS, dean's records.

The Depression and then World War II sorely tested Sturgis's administrative skills. During the Depression, painful cuts in the department were required, including reduction in salaries and dismissal of one faculty member.[61] Even with the belt tightening, Sturgis continued to lead a strong department, with Isaacs, Wilson, and Newburgh establishing themselves as accomplished researchers. With the advent of World War II, the financial emergency abated, but was replaced by a severe shortage of manpower. Virtually every able-bodied physician served in the armed services, and Sturgis had to scrounge for enough faculty simply to care for the patients and teach the students. The millions of servicemen meant a smaller population base for admittance to the hospital, and Sturgis was forced to write the dean lamenting the paucity of adequate teaching material.[62] There was, of course, little to be done to correct the situation.

As the war approached its conclusion, Sturgis recognized that a new era in American medicine was about to begin, and he sought to position the department to capitalize on it. After canvassing officers in the medical corps as a consultant to the Army, he returned to Ann Arbor committed to establishing postgraduate training for returning physicians.[63] Even more presciently, Sturgis recognized that World War II represented a watershed in the financing of medical research, predicting that after the war the federal government would become the largest supporter of medical research in the country.[64]

As predicted, after the war American medicine underwent explosive growth. The University of Michigan was typical. The opening of the Kresge Research Building in 1953 added much-needed research space, and the entire medical school embarked on a frenzy of research activity.[65] Ironically, despite Sturgis's accurate prediction that federal funds were the wave of the future in medical research, the Department of Medicine was quite slow in taking

---

61. Sturgis to Wile, June 1, 1931, box 39, folder 1931–32S, UMMS, dean's records.

62. Sturgis to Furstenberg, September 15, 1943, and December 10, 1943, box 46, folder 1943S, UMMS, dean's records.

63. Sturgis to Furstenberg, July 7, 1945, box 48, UMMS, dean's records.

64. Cyrus C. Sturgis, "The Future of Medical Research," in Frank Sladen, ed., *Psychiatry and the War* (Springfield: Charles C. Thomas, 1943), 75–93.

65. Index to UMMS collection, Bentley Library (unpublished).

advantage of the landslide of federal money.[66] This resulted from two forces.

First, departmental faculty performed little basic research. Sturgis remained wedded to an observationalist philosophy whose research credo had become unfashionable by the late 1950s. Virtually none of the medicine faculty were actively engaged in what would conventionally be considered basic research at this time. (This pattern was true not only of the Department of Medicine in general, but of the entire medical school during Furstenberg's tenure, as suggested by the few National Institutes of Health [NIH] research fellowships at Michigan.) Second, the surfeit of riches researchers had from private sources made it unnecessary to pursue NIH funding aggressively. At one point, Sturgis declined an opportunity for NIH funding because all research projects were fully funded.[67]

As the department grew, Sturgis personally remained interested in two areas of research, thyroid disease and hematology. He strongly supported research into the use of radioactive isotopes in the diagnosis and treatment of thyroid disorders. He continued to direct the Simpson Institute and its hematologists, and produced a textbook of hematology.[68] Despite these specialty interests, and the growing importance of specialization in postwar medicine, Sturgis remained first and foremost a general internist. Like Christian,[69] he was always slightly uncomfortable with specialization, noting

66. When compared to Yale, Columbia, Hopkins, Washington University, and Harvard, Michigan had the smallest number of research fellowships (one, versus three to twelve). In a comparison of projects likely to be related primarily to internal medicine—grants issued by the National Institute of Arthritis and Metabolic Disease, the National Cancer Institute, the National Institute of Allergy and Infectious Diseases, cardiology, and general research grants divisions of the NIH—Michigan also received by far the smallest amount of grant support (64 grants versus 96 to 191). U.S. Department of Health, Education, and Welfare, Public Health Service, National Institutes of Health, *Public Health Service Grants and Fellowships Awarded by the National Institutes of Health 1958*, P.H.S. Publication #624 (Washington, D.C.: U.S. Government Printing Office, 1958).

67. Sturgis to Furstenberg, May 28, 1953, box 56, folder 1953, Sl–Sz, UMMS, dean's records.

68. Cyrus C. Sturgis, *Hematology* (Springfield: Charles C. Thomas, 1947).

69. Christian to Sturgis, November 5, 1948, Sturgis family scrapbook. Upon reviewing Sturgis's textbook of hematology, Christian writes, "I have long felt that one of the best things I did at the P.B.B.H. was to insist that he who had a special interest also regularly care for patients of all sorts and so be not a specialist alone but a broad clinician interested in a specialty. I believe this is an important reason why you, Sam Levine and others have to offer in their writings something lacking in those of most."

the patient has not infrequently suffered from the narrow efficiency of specialism . . . . [a] physician may be preeminent in his own chosen field but conspicuously deficient or disinterested or both in other aspects of medicine. In my opinion the ideal situation in hematology or any other branch of internal medicine, is the practice of a specialty by a physician who has an excellent background and training in internal medicine.[70]

It comes as no surprise that the key positions that Sturgis held in professional societies were not in hematology or endocrine societies but rather as a member of the board of regents and ultimately president of the American College of Physicians.[71]

Sturgis as Teacher

As important as Sturgis's administrative accomplishments were to the department, his teaching skills were his greatest legacy. If his administrative style can be labeled humble, his teaching style might best be described as regal. The striking unanimity and force of recollections by Sturgis's former students are a tribute to his skills as a teacher. His style was that of the classic Oslerian teacher, and, although adept at lecturing, he was best in the clinical arena.[72]

Sturgis earned the devotion of his students with a combination of attributes. First was his enormous skill as a physician. Even during his earliest years, Sturgis was recognized as an outstanding clinician. This is corroborated not only by his selection by Christian as his associate in private practice, but also by the evidence that many members of the Harvard faculty had Sturgis care for their friends, family, and employees.[73] This skill was linked to an enjoyment of teaching, with a recognition of its enormous effect on students. A tough professor, Sturgis leavened his demands with a fine sense of humor. (His sons recall that he was constantly searching joke books for new material.) Building on a sensibility created by his early expe-

---

70. Sturgis, *Hematology*, x.

71. "Cyrus Cressey Sturgis," *Annals of Internal Medicine* 41 (1954): 183.

72. Interviews with Drs. William Beierwaltes, Ron Bishop, Giles Bole, William Castor, Irwin Duff, Stefan Fajans, Richard Judge, and Chris Zarafonetis, summer 1990.

73. Hans Zinsser to Sturgis, January 18, 1927, and F. W. Peabody to Sturgis, February 26, 1925, Sturgis family scrapbook.

riences with soldier's heart, Sturgis frequently lectured on the relationship between physical and mental health.[74]

Finally, Sturgis's renown as a teacher derived less from the knowledge he imparted than from the attitudes he inculcated. His teachings called students to a sense of duty and responsibility, while emphasizing a recognition that patients are more than a collection of organs.[75] He rejected overreliance on technology and insisted that diagnostic studies remain the servants of a superior history and physical performed by a physician exercising his or her critical faculties.[76]

Conclusion

The career of Cyrus Cressey Sturgis highlights the tensions that buffeted internal medicine between 1917 and 1957. As an academic discipline, internal medicine struggled to reconcile the demands of patient care, teaching, and research. The growing complexity of both medical research and medical care made this an increasingly difficult task.

Sturgis's tenure at the University of Michigan is particularly notable because the department's history defies the conventional wisdom that experimental medicine had become the only acceptable paradigm for academic internists in the post–World War II era. The faculty under Sturgis performed very little basic research and devoted considerable attention to both patient care and medical education. The research that was performed continued the observationalist tradition with an emphasis on practical, clinical problems.

The career of Cyrus Sturgis offers a model of internal medicine that existed beyond the confines of the laboratory and remained an important thread throughout the twentieth century. The election of Sturgis to high office in the American College of Physicians, and his continued leadership of a well-regarded department of medicine, demonstrate that a nonexperimentalist could play an important role in academic internal medicine.

---

74. See for example, Sturgis to Alan Gregg, April 4, 1944, box 47, folder S1944, UMMS.

75. Interview, Dr. William Castor, summer 1990.

76. See Sturgis, *Hematology*, x., and two unpublished manuscripts by Sturgis, "Dr. and Pt. Relationship" and "Some Remarks Dealing with the Art of the Practice of Medicine," Department of Internal Medicine papers, Bentley Library.

Frank Norman Wilson: Theory, Technology, and Electrocardiography

Joel D. Howell

The career of Frank Norman Wilson can best be characterized as consistent. Wilson spent most of his life at a single institution, the University of Michigan, studying a single phenomenon, the electrical activity of the human heart. He did so in ways that molded medicine and mathematics into innovative solutions to a series of technical problems. In so doing, he was able to build upon earlier attempts to record the electrical action of the human heart (fig. 9).

People have long noted that muscular contraction is associated with electrical activity.[1] The heart is a large muscle, one that for centuries has been the object of attention. Late in the nineteenth century, in London, Augustus Waller used a capillary electrometer to record the electrical action of the human heart, but his method was technically difficult and impractical for routine clinical investigation. Waller's work stimulated Willem Einthoven, in the Netherlands, to investigate other ways to record the heartbeat, and in 1902 Einthoven succeeded in devising a string galvanometer to record the electrical action of the heart, an invention that brought him a Nobel Prize in medicine or physiology in 1924.[2] However, lack of

---

1. The best general overview of ideas about electricity in living things is found in Louis N. Katz and Herman K. Hellerstein, "Electrocardiography," in Alfred P. Fishman and Dickinson W. Richards, eds., *Circulation of the Blood: Men and Ideas* (New York: Oxford University Press, 1964), 265–351.

2. For details on the history of the electrocardiogram, see George E. Burch and Nicholas P. DePasquale, *A History of Electrocardiography* (Chicago: Year Book, 1964; reprinted San Francisco: Norman Publishing, 1990); John Burnett, "The Origins of the Electrocardiograph as a Clinical Instrument," *Medical History* suppl. no. 5 (1985): 53–76.

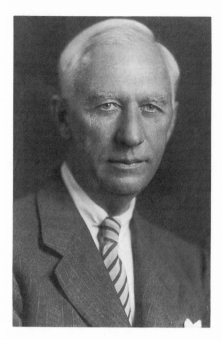

Fig. 9. Frank Norman Wilson

cooperation from clinicians limited Einthoven's clinical application of the new instrument. In 1908 Thomas Lewis, a young London physician, visited Einthoven and returned home with an electrocardiogram machine. From 1908 to about 1922, Lewis applied the new machine to the clinical study of the heart, focusing on the study of abnormal heart rhythms, or arrhythmias.[3] After Lewis, the next generation of electrocardiogram researchers studied the form, rather than the rhythm, of the electrical record of the heartbeat. Frank Norman Wilson dominated this period. He spent much of his career attempting to understand the form of the electrocardiogram and successfully applying theories of physics and mathematics to solve practical clinical problems. In so doing, he proposed technical explanations and devised technical solutions that we continue to use in the 1990s.

---

3. For discussion of Lewis's use of the machine, see Joel D. Howell, "Early Perceptions of the Electrocardiogram: From Arrhythmia to Infarction," *Bulletin of the History of Medicine* 58 (1984): 83–98.

Wilson's Early Years

The son of a farmer, Frank Wilson was born in a small, frame house in Livonia Township, Michigan, in 1890, not far from the University of Michigan, where he was to spend most of his career.[4] Wilson's mathematical skill appeared early in life; while in grade school he helped the county assessor with the tax rolls.[5] He attended Western High School from 1903 to 1907. Wilson then studied at the University of Michigan as an undergraduate and as a medical student, graduating in 1913 as a member of A.O.A., the medical school honor society. In that year he married Juel Mahoney, a student at the University of Michigan School of Music. Their only child, Julie Ann, was born in 1914.

Upon graduation from medical school in 1913, Wilson joined the Department of Internal Medicine as an assistant in charge of outpatients, for a salary of $500 per year. In that year, the department's chairman, Albion Walter Hewlett, already a well-established scholar of the cardiovascular system, purchased an electrocardiogram machine and put Wilson in charge of operating the new instrument. This was one of the earliest machines to be used in the United States. In 1909, only four years earlier, Alfred Cohn had brought the first electrocardiogram machine in the United States to New York's Mt. Sinai Hospital; the first American paper on the machine appeared in

---

4. For general biographical information on Frank Wilson, see George R. Herrmann, "An appreciation of Frank Wilson, M.D.," *American Heart Journal* 40 (1950): 647–49; Franklin D. Johnston, "Frank Norman Wilson, November 19, 1890–September 11, 1952," *Circulation* 6 (1952): 641–42; Samuel A. Levine, "A Tribute to Dr. Wilson," *University of Michigan Medical Bulletin* 18 (1952): 276–78; Ian Hill, "Frank N. Wilson," *British Heart Journal* 15 (1953): 259–60; Samuel A. Levine, "Frank Norman Wilson, 1890–1952," *Transactions of the Association of American Physicians* 56 (1953): 18–19; Louis N. Katz, "Frank Norman Wilson: Physician, Scholar, Friend," in Louis N. Katz and Arthur S. Cain, eds., *Instrumental Methods in Cardiac Diagnosis* (New York: Hoeber-Harper, 1956), 33–38; Thomas M. Durant, "Dr. Frank N. Wilson, a Biographical Sketch," *Pharos* 22 (1959): 16–23; J. K. Kahn and J. D. Howell, "Frank Norman Wilson," *Clinical Cardiology* 10 (1987): 616–18. A biographical sketch as well as a bibliography of Wilson's papers may be found in Franklin D. Johnston and Eugene Lepeschkin, eds., *Selected Papers of Dr. Frank N. Wilson* (Ann Arbor, Mich.: Edwards Brothers, 1954).

5. Fred Jenner Hodges, "Preface" to 14th Wilson Lecture in Cardiology. Bound volume of correspondence relating to the Frank Wilson Lectureship, given to Mrs. Wilson by Ted Hodges, ed., and consulted at the Stockbridge Farm. Hereafter referred to as Lecture Volume.

1910.[6] Wilson thus began his career challenged with a new and relatively untested clinical tool.

Given the newness of the machine, and the lack of respect many physicians of the period gave instrumental studies in general,[7] it was not surprising that the accommodations for this new tool and its operator were less than ideal. Tracings with the machine were recorded on photographic plates, which needed to be developed before they could be read. Wilson and the machine were installed in a former janitors' closet that had been made into a tiny laboratory and darkroom, under the stairs leading into the hospital auditorium.[8] No windows vented the chemical fumes from the darkroom solutions, and plenty of noise from people going up and down the stairs into the auditorium distracted the young physician. None of these factors contributed to Wilson's standing, and some of his colleagues referred to him as "the eccentric who plays with impractical gadgets in that hole under the stairs."[9]

Nonetheless, Wilson made some interesting observations on electrocardiographic tracings (ECGs) of patients. In 1915 he published a report on a twenty-three-year-old bookkeeper who complained of tachycardia, a rapid heartbeat, at rates up to 170 per minute. The arrhythmia would start and stop quite abruptly, and could be terminated with the drug atropine. Wilson attributed this phenomenon to vagal stimulation. He published an ECG showing a short P-R interval, which is probably the first published description of the syndrome later known as Wolf-Parkinson-White syndrome.[10] (The vagus is a

---

6. Walter B. James and Horatio B. Williams, "The Electrocardiogram in Clinical Medicine," *American Journal of the Medical Sciences* 140 (1910): 408–21. Cohn soon left Mt. Sinai for the Rockefeller Institute, where he enjoyed a distinguished career.

7. Gerald Geison, "Divided We Stand: Physiologists and Clinicians in the American Context," in Morris J. Vogel and Charles E. Rosenberg, eds., *The Therapeutic Revolution* (Philadelphia: University of Pennsylvania Press, 1979), 67–90.

8. Julie Wilson-Lepeschkin, "Three Cardiologists from a Mural," *Advances in Cardiology* 10 (1974): 11–17. The published version is an abridgment of a talk presented at the University of Vermont, August 1972, a seventeen-page typewritten manuscript entitled "Cardiologists I Have Known."

9. Quotation from Joel K. Kahn, "Frank Norman Wilson, M.D., and the Development of Electrocardiography," unpublished manuscript.

10. F. N. Wilson, "A Case in which the Vagus Influenced the Form of the Ventricular Complex of the Electrocardiogram," *Archives of Internal Medicine* 16 (1915): 1008–27.

major nerve in the thorax. The P-R interval measures the time between electrical activity of the atria and the ventricles, the upper and
the lower chambers of the heart.)

In 1916, Albion Hewlett left the University of Michigan to become chairman of Stanford's Department of Internal Medicine. Before he left, he arranged for Frank Wilson to move to Washington
University as an instructor in medicine, the only academic position
Wilson ever held away from the University of Michigan. There, he
joined a distinguished group of academicians, including George
Dock, who had left the University of Michigan for Tulane in 1908 and
since 1910 had been professor of medicine and dean of the medical
school, Joseph Erlanger, chairman of the department of physiology
(who was to win the Nobel Prize in medicine or physiology in 1944),
and George Canby Robinson, who conducted the course in
electrocardiography and was later to serve as dean and professor of
medicine at Vanderbilt. All in all, it offered a strong working environment and opportunities for advancement that were, in Hewlett's
opinion, superior to those Wilson left behind in Ann Arbor.[11]

War Work: Contacts with Lewis and Einthoven

Wilson had been at Washington University a little over a year when,
in 1917, he received a telegram from the United States Surgeon General asking him to join a group of U.S. Army physicians working in
Colchester, England. There, a distinguished group of physicians
were studying a disease known variously as DAH (for disordered
action of the heart), soldier's heart, or, later, the effort syndrome.
The disease was characterized by breathlessness, palpitations, and a
sense of overwhelming dread no doubt common (and appropriate)
among many of the soldiers on the Western Front. The syndrome
was of far more than merely academic interest. It was a major cause
of loss of manpower, the third most common cause of discharge from
the British Army. The war had led to an extremely unpopular draft,
and official attention focused on ways of reducing the numbers of
additional men that would need to be inducted into the Army. Al-

---

11. Hewlett to Wilson, June 24, 1916, quoted in Wilson-Lepeschkin, "Cardiologists I Have Known."

though a far less common reason for disability among soldiers than wounds and injuries, men with heart disease appeared to constitute a group with whom physicians stood a reasonable chance of success in returning the men to the front. Wilson worked with this research group from October 1917 to January 1919.[12]

The research team concluded that soldier's heart probably did not result from intrinsic cardiac disease. Moreover, they designed a program that was somewhat successful in returning soldiers to the battlefield. But for Frank Wilson, as important as the solutions to the problem at hand were the people with whom he formed lasting and instructive relationships.[13] Most important was his relationship with Thomas Lewis of London, later knighted for his work on soldier's heart. The leader of the group's research effort, Lewis was at that time the world's leading expert on the interpretation of the electrocardiogram. He and Einthoven were the first two of the triumvirate of great electrocardiographers; Wilson would become the third. Lewis and Wilson respected each other as scientists and enjoyed each other as friends. When work slowed at Colchester, Lewis showed Wilson the English countryside and introduced him to bird photography. Wilson continued to enjoy that hobby for the rest of his life, buying new cameras and lenses and delighting in taking photographs of a wide range of birds (fig. 10).[14]

In 1919 Wilson returned to St. Louis, where he assumed responsibility for the heart station and for all patients with heart disease. A year later, in 1920, Dean Victor Vaughan was able to recruit Wilson to return to the University of Michigan, where he remained on staff for the next thirty-two years.

---

12. For discussion of what this group did, and how that relates to the history of British cardiology, see Joel D. Howell, "'Soldier's Heart': The Redefinition of Heart Disease and Specialty Formation in Early Twentieth-Century Great Britain," *Medical History* supplement no. 5 (1985): 34–52.

13. Charles F. Wooley, "From Irritable Heart to Mitral Valve Prolapse—World War I, the British Experience and Thomas Lewis," *American Journal of Cardiology* 58 (1986): 844–49; Charles F. Wooley, "From Irritable Heart to Mitral Valve Prolapse: World War I. The U.S. Experience and the Origin of Neurocirculatory Asthenia," *American Journal of Cardiology* 59 (1987): 1183–86.

14. Wilson consistently comments on bird photographs in his letters to Lewis. For example, November 10, 1925 and September 23, 1929. Thomas Lewis papers in the Contemporary Medical Archives Centre of the Wellcome Institute of the History of Medicine, London. Hereafter referred to as Lewis papers.

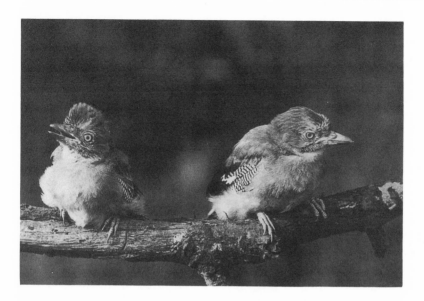

Fig. 10. An example of Wilson's skill at bird photography

Wilson's Return to Ann Arbor

Wilson returned to Ann Arbor in the middle of an important time for the University. The medical center had recently adopted a plan under which all of the medical staff worked full-time for the university. The old Catherine Street hospital had become overcrowded, and in 1917 the state legislature appropriated funds for a new hospital, $1,000,000 to be provided in three yearly installments. War intervened, and construction finally started in 1920, the year that Wilson came back. By 1921 the outer shell of the hospital was completed, but all of the appropriated funds were gone. The new hospital sat boarded up until an additional appropriation of $2,300,000 in 1923 allowed it to be completed.[15] Finally, in August of 1925, 597 patients moved into the new hospital, a new hospital that, as we shall see, Wilson had specifically equipped to pursue his research agenda.

Between 1920 and 1925, Wilson made do with suboptimal conditions. Nonetheless, his work was well received, and the number of

15. Wilfred B. Shaw, ed., *The University of Michigan: An Encyclopedic Survey* (Ann Arbor: University of Michigan Press, 1952).

patients on whom an ECG was requested steadily increased. Wilson was able to hire an assistant and engage two interns in order to free him from routine work. The institution charged from $5 to $25 for a tracing, depending upon the patient's ability to pay. There was no charge for ECGs taken for the purposes of teaching or research, areas in which Wilson spent increasing amounts of time.

Wilson's observations reveal a gradual shift in his interests. The 1915 publication discussed above, fairly typical of most early reports on the ECG, was about cardiac rhythm abnormalities. Most reports of that genre described characteristic patterns of the heartbeat, based on the rhythm of excitation of the upper and lower cardiac chambers.[16] Those patterns were related to well-known physiological patterns that had been worked out by direct observations in animals and by study of the pulse waves in human beings. Wilson's primary contributions, however, were to come from moving the electrocardiogram to a new area of investigation, the study of the form of the complexes, rather than their rhythm. Einthoven had defined the three primary complexes. The P wave reflects electrical action of the upper cardiac chambers, the atria. The QRS complex represents depolarization of the lower cardiac chambers, the ventricles, while the T wave represents repolarization of those chambers. Wilson wrote a brief report in 1923, which documents that drinking ice water could cause the last wave of the ECG complex, the T wave, to invert.[17] This convinced Wilson of the lability of T-wave changes, and throughout his subsequent career Wilson discouraged physicians from placing too much emphasis on the T wave. The report also marks a shift from Wilson's study of rhythm to his study of the form of the waves.

Although still young, Wilson drew to Ann Arbor the only two people working on electrocardiography on a level comparable to his own. Thomas Lewis, by then Sir Thomas Lewis, visited in 1922. Although Lewis received an honorary D.Sc. from the University of Michigan, many suspected that the real reason for Sir Thomas's visit was to photograph a bird no longer found in Europe, the black tern. No doubt Wilson enjoyed both events.

---

16. See Howell, "Early Use of the Electrocardiogram," and Joel D. Howell, *Machines' Meanings: British and American Use of Medical Technology, 1890–1930* (Ph.D. dissertation, University of Pennsylvania, Philadelphia, 1987).

17. F. N. Wilson and Russel Finch, "The Effect of Drinking Iced Water upon the Form of the T Deflection of the Electrocardiogram," *Heart* 10 (1923): 275–78.

In 1924 Willem Einthoven came to Ann Arbor. Although they corresponded often, this was the only time that Wilson and Einthoven met. The meeting came at an important time for Einthoven, for he continued his trip to Boston, where he found that for his invention of the electrocardiograph he had been awarded the 1924 Nobel Prize. During the visit, Einthoven and Wilson dashed off a friendly postcard to their fellow electrocardiographer, Thomas Lewis.[18] Einthoven also discussed with Wilson a new machine, a double-string galvanometer.

A New Machine, a New Hospital, a New Set of Intellectual Tools

The heart of Einthoven's original invention was the string galvanometer, a tiny filament suspended between the poles of an electromagnet that moved in response to an electrical signal. The machine used a single filament, and recorded a single line. A new machine, the double-string galvanometer, was to play an important role in Wilson's revision of ideas about the electrocardiograph and the tracings it created. The double-string galvanometer could simultaneously record two leads of the electrocardiogram, projecting together the image of two strings. To analyze arrhythmias, the goal of the previous generation of electrocardiographers, one needed only to separate the action of the upper and the lower cardiac chambers. For this purpose, a single lead sufficed; by sequentially taking different leads one could obtain the information thought necessary at that time. But to accomplish what Wilson desired, to work out the theory of the QRS complex, one needed to record more than one lead simultaneously. By so doing, one could plot the precise vector of the heart's electrical action.

The mere existence of the instrument did not dictate such a use. Thomas Lewis, too, used a double-string galvanometer. But Lewis chose to use the second string to record not another lead of the ECG, but heart sounds, a phonocardiogram. This choice was entirely consistent with a different approach to the instrument, a different agenda for the questions it should answer. Lewis worked within an

---

18. H. A. Snellen, *Two Pioneers of Electrocardiography* (Rotterdam: Donker Academic Publications, 1983), 118.

English tradition of medicine that placed physical diagnosis at the center of medical diagnosis. Wilson, though, was far less concerned with physical diagnosis and far more willing to invest authority in the machine.

Early in 1924, Wilson started to pursue the funds necessary for the double-string galvanometer.[19] When he failed initially to obtain authorization to purchase the machine, he approached the problem in a familiar, classic, academic fashion—he threatened to take another job. In this case the other job was at Vanderbilt, where his old friend and colleague from Washington University, George Canby Robinson, had recently been appointed professor and dean. Wilson made this other opportunity known to the University of Michigan Medical School dean, Hugh Cabot. The dean wrote Richard Burton, the president of the University. Burton replied the very next day that although the regents, of course, had the final say, at least he and one regent would "urge favorable action" on Wilson's request.[20] Wilson later used Einthoven's visit to expedite approval for the machine. Wilson was eventually promised $4,000 for "special equipment," the double-string galvanometer, with lenses custom-made by the Carl Zeis Company.[21] The equipment was quite explicitly understood as part of what would be necessary in the new hospital to carry on electrocardiographic studies of heart disease, a relatively new concept for academic medical investigators.

In 1925, the new hospital opened, and Wilson and his colleagues moved into a brand-new, eleven-room "heart station."[22] The concept of a heart station was important for people wishing to study heart disease using instrumental apparatus, such as the electrocardiogram machine. It aided professionalization by gathering together in one place those who wished to carry on such research, as well as providing a place of employment for practitioners wishing to learn how to

19. Wilson to (Dean Hugh) Cabot, October 14, 1924, mentions discussions in January of that year. In University of Michigan Medical School papers, box 35, dean's correspondence files, Michigan Historical Collections, Ann Arbor. Hereafter referred to as UMMS papers.

20. Hugh Cabot to (President) Richard Burton, March 4, 1924; Burton to Cabot, March 5, 1924, UMMS papers.

21. Wilson to Cabot, October 14, 1924, UMMS papers.

22. Frank N. Wilson and Paul S. Barker, "The Heart Station of the University of Michigan Hospital," reprint from *Methods and Problems of Medical Education*, 18th series (New York: Rockefeller Foundation, 1930).

use the machines. Organizations such as the American Heart Association, which would later come to define who cardiologists are and what they do, were more interested in public health than in physiological instruments and had given scant attention to Wilson and his colleagues. The heart station at the new hospital provided a symbolic gathering point for a small number of researchers. It also provided a way to integrate clinical and research activities. Shortly before the move to the new hospital, Wilson had used the increasing numbers of patients being sent for an electrocardiogram to convince the dean to provide for additional staff, to assign medical house officers to his team, and to provide a pay raise for his assistant.[23] Without a special place to put the instrument, it would not have been so easy to establish the need for additional staff to carry on research and clinical programs.

Heart stations also had immediate practical value. They were places to put big and bulky equipment. The heart station in the new, 1925 hospital went a step further. The entire hospital was wired for the recording of electrocardiograms.[24] Since wires from the heart station went to every ward, patients did not need to be wheeled down to the heart station, nor did the cumbrous galvanometer need to be taken to their beds. One, two, or three leads could be recorded. A private telephone service provided direct communication between the wards, private rooms, or operating room, and the galvanometer room. The hospital itself thus aided the taking of ECGs and the pursuit of Wilson's research agenda.

1927

The year 1927 marked an important turning point in Wilson's career for many reasons. First, the double-string galvanometer arrived, giving him the use of a machine better for his purposes than almost any other in the world. Second, administrative changes in the Depart-

---

23. Wilson to Cabot, December 20, 1924; Cabot's reply, December 24, 1924. It is worthy of note that a special nurse was requested for the heart station, specifically to prepare "private female patients" for examination, UMMS papers.

24. Einthoven had recorded ECGs at a distance, too. However, Einthoven had a single connection, devoted primarily to research. Michigan's new hospital, one of the largest university hospitals, completely wired for taking electrocardiograms, was a major innovation.

ment of Internal Medicine promised Wilson a much-improved working environment. Wilson had been recruited in 1920 by the dean, Victor Vaughan. Louis Newburgh was then acting head of the department, but without control over the budget or the privilege of making new appointments. Newburgh was followed as chair by Louis Warfield (1922–25), who left on unfavorable terms. Then quickly followed Preston Hickey, a professor of roentgenology, and James Bruce, recruited from private practice in Saginaw. In other words, Wilson had worked from 1920 to 1927 under a series of short-lived appointments held by relatively weak administrators. Unstable conditions made Wilson's scientific work difficult; some of his most valued associates left the department because of the weak leadership. When Wilson was asked to consider the job of department head himself, Sir Thomas Lewis advised him to accept and to deal with the situation "ruthlessly."[25] Wilson, however, declined, possibly because he did not want to devote time to administration.

The 1927 improvement for the Department of Internal Medicine was in large part a product of private philanthropy. In 1923, Mrs. Thomas Henry Simpson, the widow of a Detroit industrialist, had given almost $500,000 to the University of Michigan to found an institute for research on diseases of the blood as a memorial to her husband. The Simpson Memorial Institute was finished by 1926, and Cyrus Sturgis was recruited to head the Institute in 1927. The next year, James Bruce was made chair of the newly created Department of Postgraduate Medicine, and Sturgis was named chairman of Internal Medicine; he remained for thirty years, until 1958. In his first year, Sturgis made one of his most insightful decisions. He reorganized the medical services, combining cardiology and metabolism with general medicine, to give Newburgh and Wilson increased time for research. It is probably not a coincidence that, in the decade following Sturgis's appointment, Wilson accomplished some of his most significant work.

But all did not go well for Wilson in 1927. He suffered for some time from a poorly defined but debilitating illness. Eventually, his gallbladder was removed, but he required a prolonged convalescence. To have a quiet place to recuperate, the Wilsons bought a farm

25. Lewis to Wilson, October 24, 1924, quoted in Wilson-Lepeschkin, "Cardiologists I Have Known."

outside of Stockbridge, Michigan. There, Frank Wilson slowly recovered, in a peaceful, relaxed environment—no electricity, no plumbing—thirty-six miles away from the noise and heat of the city. The farm was to play an important role in Wilson's life, to be the site of many informal gatherings of his friends and collaborators, and to be central to much of his personal and professional life.

Wilson took advantage of the inactivity forced on him by his illness to study mathematics, a field that he had decided was central to understanding the ECG. His interest in mathematics had started around 1914, when, as he recalled, he

> realized that in order to do worthwhile work in electrocardiography I ought to know the principles that govern the flow of electricity in volume conductors. I found that to understand these principles and apply them I must have a greater knowledge of mathematics than I possessed at that time. I therefore bought a book on analytic geometry and one on the calculus and have studied mathematics on and off ever since.[26]

During his convalescence, Wilson studied higher algebra, analytic geometry, and calculus, and he came back to work with a new set of intellectual tools to complement the new physical tools of the double-string galvanometer.[27]

Bundle-Branch Block

Wilson's first major advance had to do with understanding the form of the electrocardiographic tracing that results when part of the specialized conduction system of the heart fails to work properly, a con-

---

26. Typewritten pages, no title, starting, "This was dictated to Julie Wilson Lepeschkin by her father, Frank Norman Wilson in the summer of 1952 . . . . " The two books noted were Ziwet and Hopkins, *Analytic Geometry*, and Davis, *Calculus*. (Alexander Ziwet and Louis Allen Hopkins, *Analytic Geometry and Principles of Algebra* (New York: Macmillan, 1913); Ellery Williams Davis and William Charles Brenke, *The Calculus* (New York: Macmillan, 1912). Both of these books went through several editions, both before and after the period when Wilson most likely first looked at them. Wilson noted that he later made extensive use of Mellor, *Higher Mathematics for Students of Physics and Chemistry* (presumably, Joseph William Mellor, *Higher Mathematics for Students of Chemistry and Physics* [London and New York: Longman's Green, 1902]).

27. Samuel A. Levine, "Foreword" (to a special issue of the journal), *Circulation* 2 (1950): 3–4.

dition called bundle-branch block. In 1909, Eppinger and Rothberger had recognized the specialized nature of specific conducting tissues in the heart. They showed that destroying a small part of the ventricular septum of a dog's heart, first with silver nitrate, later with a knife, produced more of an effect on the form of the ECG than destroying much larger parts of the left ventricle, the major cardiac chamber.[28] The ECG, recorded with retroesophageal leads (leads placed behind the heart, in the esophagus), showed a widening of the QRS complex. They speculated that the effect resulted from injury to specialized conduction tissues running in the part of the heart that they had destroyed. In 1910, Eppinger and Stoerk reported a similar ECG in a thirty-five-year-old man with heart failure. Since they assumed that the retroesophageal lead in dogs was analogous to lead III in human beings, and since both the dog's and the man's tracings were primarily negative, Eppinger and Rothberger concluded, by analogy with the results of injuring the right bundle in dogs, that the man suffered from right-bundle-branch block.

Thomas Lewis carried on further experiments. By damaging the conduction tissues of a dog he was able to produce alternating right- and left-bundle-branch block. He concluded that the main deflection in right-bundle-branch block was up in lead I and down in lead III, with the reverse for left-bundle-branch block. In 1921, Wilson agreed in public that the question was basically closed, that "The conclusions arrived at . . . are so fortified on every side that it is improbable that they will need material revision."[29] However, in private, Wilson was not so sure. The preceding year he had mentioned to Lewis two cases of bundle-branch block in which "the lesions found at autopsy are on the wrong side." Wilson went on to suggest that "the right ventricle might be stimulated during a thoracic operation and the form of the resulting extrasystole would settle the question, once [and] for all."[30] Nine years later, Wilson was to have the opportunity to do just that.

In 1929, while Wilson was still slowly recuperating, three of his

28. Arthur Hollman, "The History of Bundle Branch Block," *Medical History* supplement no. 5 (1985): 82–102.

29. Frank N. Wilson and George R. Herrmann, "An Experimental Study of Incomplete Bundle Branch Block and of the Refractory Period of the Heart of the Dog," *Heart* 8 (1921): 229–96.

30. Wilson to Lewis, May 7, 1920, Lewis papers.

colleagues at the University of Michigan grasped an opportunity to ascertain for certain the ECG patterns in bundle-branch block. A thirty-year-old man with lobar pneumonia had developed strep viridans pericarditis (a bacterial infection of the heart's lining). As was common before the availability of antibiotics, a pericardiostomy— surgical creation of a hole in the pericardium—allowed the wound to drain. For the next twenty-one days, the patient's heart lay open to the outside world. During that time, Paul S. Barker, A. Garrard Macleod, and John Alexander stimulated each ventricle directly from the surface of the heart. They recorded the ECG effects of such stimulation simultaneously in two leads, taking advantage of both the double-string galvanometer and the hospital's wiring system that allowed them to record the electrical action of the heart without having to move the patient to the heart station. Unfortunately, the patient died the day after the wound was closed. However, pathological examination of his heart verified that the only cardiac problem was pericarditis; there was no intrinsic cardiac disease.

The electrocardiographic tracings revealed that the previously accepted patterns of bundle-branch block were exactly reversed. Because the physicians had directly stimulated each ventricle in turn, there could be no mistake about the side of the heart from which the impulse came. These results were so startling and important that Wilson tried to publish the findings in *Heart,* the journal founded and edited by Sir Thomas Lewis. Their correspondence on this issue reveals a rather heated exchange of views between two leaders of the field.

Lewis initially characterized the findings as "off the ordinary lines, and puzzling," and questioned the authors at length as to exactly how they had located the points on the heart.[31] Wilson carefully explained the process. He noted that he shared Lewis's hesitancy in accepting the results, that he, too, was "rather reluctant to believe that our current views were upside down," but that either the particular patient was a "striking exception" or that the previous views were wrong. "This [latter] conclusion is troublesome," Wilson said, "but I am afraid it is inescapable."[32]

Lewis replied rather testily. He outlined the changes necessary

---

31. Lewis to Wilson, October 4, 1929, Lewis papers.
32. Wilson to Lewis, October 18, 1929, Lewis papers.

before he would publish the paper, changes that would, in essence, retract the central findings of the Michigan paper. Wilson responded in detail to each of the points Lewis raised. He left Lewis "distinctly shaken, though as yet unconvinced."[33] Nonetheless, Lewis eventually agreed to publish the paper without major alterations.

However, early in 1930, Lewis reversed himself. Because a preliminary version of the study had been presented to the Association of American Physicians and a summary had been published in their *Transactions*, Lewis asserted that he could not publish the full paper in *Heart*.[34] Wilson reluctantly sent the paper to the *American Heart Journal*. He was not himself an author on the full publication of these findings, a pattern of allowing others to take the lead in publishing that no doubt led to increased loyalty among his collaborators.[35] Wilson did, the next year, publish a detailed account of the technical problems that had led his friend Sir Thomas Lewis astray.[36]

New Ideas, New ECG Leads

Stimulated by the bundle-branch block findings, Wilson set out to develop a clinically useful way of recording the electrical action taking place under an electrode. To accomplish this goal, he needed to devise a new technique for recording the electrocardiogram. Einthoven's original three leads had each recorded the potential difference between two limbs. This difference, however, was not what Wilson needed. He wanted instead to use a semidirect electrode,

---

33. Wilson to Lewis, November 25, 1929; Lewis to Wilson, December 6, 1929, Lewis papers.

34. Paul S. Barker, A. Garrard Macleod, John Alexander, and Frank N. Wilson, "The Excitatory Process Observed in the Exposed Human Heart," *Transactions of the Association of American Physicians* 44 (1929): 125–33. The positions of the two men are summarized in Wilson to Lewis, January 30, 1930, and Lewis to Wilson, February 8, 1930, Lewis papers.

35. The publication was Paul S. Barker, A. Garrard Macleod and John Alexander, "The Excitatory Process Observed in the Exposed Human Heart," *American Heart Journal* 5 (1930): 720–42. Wilson's generous habits with regards to publication are noted by Hill, "Frank Wilson," and by the listing of "28 Papers from Doctor Wilson's Laboratory to which He Contributed without Appearing as Co-Author," in Johnston and Lepeschkin, *Selected Papers:* xliv–xlvi.

36. Frank N. Wilson, A. Garrard Macleod, and Paul S. Barker, "The Interpretation of the Initial Deflections of the Ventricular Complex of the Electrocardiogram," *American Heart Journal* 6 (1931): 637–65.

analogous to the direct electrodes that his colleagues placed directly on the heart of the patient described above, to record electrical action at a single point rather than the electrical difference between two locations. Obviously, direct recording from the human heart is usually impractical in clinical care, but Wilson believed that important clinical information could be obtained from a semidirect recording.

This belief led Wilson to study in some depth the underlying principles of electrocardiography. After learning the necessary mathematics, mostly on his own, he turned next to what physiologists had to say about the electrical actions of tissues. Most descriptions were not relevant to clinical medicine. Standard physiological theory was derived from experiments on isolated muscle strips surrounded by a nonconducting medium. The human heart, however, was neither an isolated muscle strip, nor surrounded by a nonconducting medium. The heart is a current generator in a bounded-volume conductor, where the boundaries are the surface of the body.

Wilson explored how the results might be different for the heart, a large and complex muscle surrounded by a nonhomogeneous thorax and bounded by an irregular body. His answer came in a long, theoretical paper on the distribution of currents produced by excitable tissues in volume conductors like the human body, a paper rejected by several journals on the grounds that it was too long and too mathematical.[37] It was finally published in abbreviated form by the *Journal of General Physiology* and in full by the University of Michigan Press as a 1933 monograph.[38] The highly technical paper disagreed with standard dogma in several respects, most notably by showing that an injured region of the heart was not an indifferent point and by proposing a dipole theory to explain the genesis of the ECG. Most important, the theory helped Wilson start to devise a practical mechanism for obtaining a unipolar, semidirect recording.

37. The paper was rejected by the *American Journal of Physiology*, the *Journal of General Physiology*, the *Journal of Cellular and Comparative Physiology*, and the *Proceedings of the Royal Society*. It was considered for publication by the Rockefeller Institute, but lack of funds due to the economic climate prevented this. See Wilson to Lewis, July 7, 1932, and Lewis to Wilson, July 29, 1932, Lewis papers.

38. F. N. Wilson, A. G. Macleod, and P. S. Barker, "The Distribution of the Action Currents Produced by Heart Muscle and Other Excitable Tissues Immersed in Extensive Conducting Media," *Journal of General Physiology* 16 (1933): 423–56; F. N. Wilson, A. G. Macleod, and P. S. Barker, *The Distribution of the Currents of Action and Injury Displayed by Heart Muscle and Other Excitable Tissues* (Ann Arbor: University of Michigan Studies, Scientific Series, vol. 18, 1933).

To record the electrical action of a point on or above the heart, Wilson wanted to place the electrode on the chest; that is, to take a precordial lead. He was not the first to put leads on the chest. Because Waller's instrument was not sensitive enough to record currents unless it was placed close to the heart, he had used a precordial lead for his 1887 demonstration. But with Einthoven's 1902 invention of the electrocardiogram, based on a much more sensitive measuring device, the string galvanometer, there was no longer any need to have the patient undress to place a lead on the chest. Almost all early ECG work was done using the leads I, II, and III as originally described by Einthoven, leads that recorded a potential difference between two points on the patient's extremities. There appeared to be no reason to attempt other combinations or locations of leads.

While Wilson was working out theory, other physicians started to apply the available tools empirically to clinical work. In 1932, Charles Wolferth and Francis Wood, in Philadelphia, showed that recording an ECG tracing from the chest could have significant clinical utility. After recording the traditional lead III, they simply took the electrode from the patient's left arm and placed it over the apex of the heart. They called this tracing lead IV. For the patient in question, it revealed—where Einthoven leads I, II, and III had not—the presence of an acute myocardial infarction, a finding of significant clinical utility.[39]

Following this demonstration, physicians started putting leads in many places. The human chest offered many options for placing an electrode, and there was no consistency or consensus about where it was best to record a tracing. Nor was there agreement on which lead system to use, or even whether an upward deflection of the tracing ought to record a positive or a negative current. Investigators carried on heated debates as to which was the superior system.

All of the leads initially used were, like Einthoven's original device, bipolar leads, recording the potential difference between two points. One electrode was placed on the chest, one placed on some distant or "indifferent" point, such as an arm or a leg. Wilson's theoretical analysis demonstrated a problem with this approach. Rather than reflecting only the electrical activation of the heart under one

---

39. Charles C. Wolferth and Francis Clark Wood, "The Electrocardiographic Diagnosis of Coronary Occlusion by the Use of Chest Leads," *American Journal of the Medical Sciences* 183 (1932): 30–35.

electrode, the tracing was also influenced by the potential at the other electrode. In other words, the supposedly indifferent electrode wasn't. To record only the electrical activity taking place under the electrode on the chest, Wilson needed to create a zero reference point against which to measure the potential of the chest electrode.

Since some electrical activity is always present, there is no true "zero" reference point in the body. But based on mathematical theory, Wilson hypothesized that he could create one by linking the three leads used for traditional tracings. Using trial and error to come up with the best resistors to put into the circuit, Wilson produced a zero reference point. Paired with an electrode on the chest, it would allow the electrode placed over the heart to record only the electrical activity of the heart, underneath the exploring electrode, unaffected by electrical action in other parts of the body. Wilson's 1934 invention was called the central terminal (fig. 11).[40] Originally put together in Wilson's laboratory, it has since been incorporated into standard practice and is used daily in tens of thousands of electrocardiogram machines around the world.[41] It provides a mechanism for recording unipolar views of the heart. This gave rise to the six precordial leads, which offer a different way of looking at the heart.

Simply having the technology available did not guarantee that clinicians would use the new leads. Procedures had to be standardized. Because so many lead systems were described in the 1930s, the publications on chest leads were characterized as "boring, difficult to read and understand, and . . . apparently [of] little value."[42] As a result, many clinicians simply ignored chest leads. Before they could be widely accepted, clinicians had to agree on how to take the leads and what they meant. The first question related to the polarity of the leads, what an upward deflection should signify. The prevailing convention was that an upward deflection indicated a negative potential. Wilson was opposed to this on the grounds of basic mathematics, and

40. F. N. Wilson, F. D. Johnson, A. G. Macleod, and P. S. Barker, "Electrocardiograms that Represent the Potential Variations of a Single Electrode," *American Heart Journal* 9 (1934): 447–58.

41. Charles E. Kossmann, "Unipolar Electrocardiography of Wilson: A Half Century Later," *American Heart Journal* 110 (1985): 901–4. For discussion of the debates over its validity, see Katz and Hellerstein, "Electrocardiography."

42. G. E. Burch, "History of Precordial Leads in Electrocardiography," *European Journal of Cardiology* 8 (1978): 207–36.

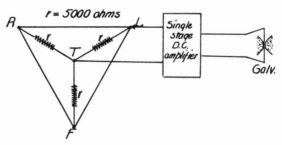

Fig. 1.—Diagram illustrating the method of leading used to record the potential variations of a single electrode. Electrodes on the right arm (*R*), left arm (*L*), and left leg (*F*) are connected through equal resistances of 5,000 ohms to a central terminal (*T*). The central terminal and an exploring electrode, or one of the extremity electrodes as indicated here, are connected to the input terminals of a vacuum-tube amplifier with a balanced plate circuit in which the string galvanometer is inserted.

Fig. 11. Wilson's "central terminal." (Reprinted from Frank N. Wilson et al., "Electrocardiograms That Represent the Potential Variations of Single Electrode," *American Heart Journal* 9, no. 4 (1934): 447.

because it was "inconsistent with the well established conventions of coordinate geometry." In 1938 Wilson served on a joint United States–Great Britain Committee that established the conventions used to denote polarity.[43] It remained only to determine where the precordial leads should be placed; these conventions also came from Frank Wilson's laboratory.[44] We now use six standard precordial leads, labeled V1 through V6.

The exploring electrode that was connected to the central terminal could be placed not only on the chest, but also on the limbs. At first these electrodes were placed on the right arm, left arm, and left foot, and these leads were then called VR, VL, and VF, after the

---

43. Arlie R. Barnes, Harold E. B. Pardee, Paul D. White, Frank N. Wilson, Charles C. Wolferth, D. Evan Bedford, John Cowan, A. N. Drury, I. G. W. Hill, John Parkinson, and P. H. Wood, "Standardization of Precordial Leads, Joint Recommendations of the American Heart Association and the Cardiac Society of Great Britain and Ireland," *American Heart Journal* 15 (1938): 107–8; Arlie R. Barnes, Harold E. B. Pardee, Paul D. White, Frank N. Wilson, Charles C. Wolferth, "Standardization of Precordial Leads: Supplementary Report," *American Heart Journal* 15 (1938): 235–39.

44. Charles E. Kossman and Franklin D. Johnston, "The Precordial Electrocardiogram. I. The Potential Variations of the Precordium and of the Extremities in Normal Subjects," *American Heart Journal* 10 (1935): 925–41.

terminology for V leads of the chest. Because of their great distance from the chest, such leads produced relatively small waves. By removing the electrode of the central terminal from the limb on which the exploring electrode was placed, the amplitude of the tracing could be increased. The "augmented" leads were labeled aVR, aVL, and aVF.[45] These three new leads, together with the six precordial leads and Einthoven's three original leads, now make up the standard twelve-lead electrocardiogram. Although it took time, eventually this system became the norm. As late as the 1950s, only Einthoven leads I, II, and III were taken routinely at the University of Michigan.[46]

Theory and Practice

Wilson made seminal contributions to our understanding of coronary artery disease. His mathematical analysis of the QRS complex explained how myocardial infarction (heart attack) produces Q waves.[47] Wilson also worked out how patterns of injury could be inferred by the pattern of Q waves in the various leads.[48] Following up on his earlier work, he explained the transient nature of T-wave changes, as opposed to the longer-lasting QRS changes.[49]

In 1941 Wilson reported what is probably an early recognition of coronary spasm, a subject that later, with the advent of coronary arteriography, became the focus of intense study.[50] As an early ex-

45. S. L. Barron, *The Development of the Electrocardiograph* (London, Cambridge Instrument Company, 1952).

46. Leon Ostrander, personal communication, July 1987.

47. Q waves are an initial negative deflection in the portion of the tracing that reflects activation of the lower cardiac chambers, the ventricles.

48. The theoretical basis of this analysis is complex. Its history has been the subject of some controversy, particularly regarding the role of Lewis, Einthoven, Wilson, and W. H. Craib and the doublet-dipole theory. See R. D. Pruitt, "Doublets, Dipoles and the Negativity Hypothesis: An Historical Note on W. H. Craib and His Relationship with F. N. Wilson and Thomas Lewis," *Johns Hopkins Medical Journal* 138 (1976): 279–88 and W. H. Craib, "For the Amusement of Cardiologists," *Perspectives in Biology and Medicine* 22 (1979): 205–31.

49. Wilson summarized his theoretical work quite readably in "The Form of the Electrocardiogram," in (Piersol) *Cyclopedia of Medicine* (Philadelphia: F. A. Davis, 1935), 3: 402–24.

50. F. N. Wilson and F. D. Johnston, "The Occurrence in Angina Pectoris of Electrocardiographic Changes Similar in Magnitude and in Kind to Those Produced by Myocardial Infarction," *American Heart Journal* 22 (1941): 64–74; J. Willis Hurst, "Coronary Spasm as Viewed by Wilson and Johnston in 1941," *American Journal of Cardiology* 57 (1986): 1000–1002.

ample of a stress test, Wilson asked a fifty-year-old man with chest pain to smoke two cigarettes, and observed changes in the man's ECG tracing characteristic of myocardial ischemia. Theory at that time held that angina (chest pain from coronary artery disease) was always due to an increase in work. Wilson said

> When . . . pronounced electrocardiographic changes of the kind produced by temporary occlusion of a large coronary artery occur, disappear, and then reappear without any material increase in heart rate or in blood pressure, this view [that angina is always due to an increase in work] is clearly untenable. It must, we think, be admitted that in some instances anginal paroxysms are precipitated by contraction of the coronary arteries involved.

Without a coronary arteriogram, Wilson could only speculate, but his speculation has since been supported by new technology.

Wilson was also active in the development of yet another way to examine the form of the ventricular complex. Always interested in the spatial orientation of the electrical action of the heart, Wilson researched ways to derive a vector representation of the excitation wave. In 1936 and 1937 three different groups, including Wilson's, independently described the use of the cathode ray terminal to record the electrical action. Wilson's group suggested the name "vectorcardiogram," which came to be the term used to describe the technique. Though popular for a time, the vectorcardiogram by the 1990s has virtually disappeared, perhaps replaced by other kinds of diagnostic technologies.[51]

Wilson at Home

Since meeting Thomas Lewis in England during World War I, Wilson had enjoyed not only photographing but also studying birds, coming

---

51. Though one should hesitate, at least momentarily, before assigning a definite relationship of cause and effect as an explanation for the disappearance of the vectorcardiogram from clinical medicine. The fine-detailed history of the vectorcardiogram could prove an interesting window into different ideas about the heart and disease. A start has been provided by George E. Burch, "The History of Vectorcardiography," *Medical History* supplement no. 5 (1985): 103–31.

to the public defense of species that he felt were unfairly attacked, such as the marsh hawk.[52] After buying the farm in Stockbridge, he converted it into a wildlife sanctuary that persisted even after his death.

The farm was central to much of Wilson's life. He used it to pursue his fascination with astronomy. He purchased a seven-inch refractor telescope from New York City, which he assembled in 1939 and he soon had an observatory made to protect it from the elements. Another example of Wilson's mathematical bent was his fascination with the motions of the heavenly bodies. He would calculate the time of some planetary event, such as when the fourth moon of Jupiter would enter eclipse. He might then insist that those assembled at a party, happily gathered singing around the piano, accompany him out to the telescope to observe the phenomenon.[53]

Wilson's power of concentration was enormous, legendary among those who told (and tell) stories about him. His daughter characterized him as an "absent-minded professor," and there are many examples of that trait. Typical is the tale of a visit to his good friend Samuel Levine, in Boston. At a party Levine hosted in Wilson's honor, Wilson went upstairs to change and failed to return. Some time later, Levine found that Wilson, engrossed in a problem, had completely forgotten about the party downstairs. When Wilson started to take off his clothes, he had assumed he was going to bed and had retired for the evening.[54]

Another example comes from the 1949 wedding of his only child, Julie Ann, to Eugene Lepeschkin, another important leader in the field of electrocardiography. The ceremony was held at the Stockbridge farm.[55] Because Wilson was ill, he remained inside, on the sofa, but with a view of the wedding, which was held under an apple

52. "Defender Turns up for the Marsh Hawk," *Detroit News* February 17, 1929.

53. Reminiscences by Ted Hodges, reported in *Wildlife Sanctuary Bulletin*, 3 (1977): 25–26. Typewritten manuscript, kindly made available by Irene Turner, edited by Julie Wilson-Lepeschkin.

54. Wilson-Lepeschkin, "Three Cardiologists," 15.

55. Wilson's quite positive feelings about his son-in-law as a scientist were expressed in his "Foreword" to Eugene Lepeschkin, *Modern Electrocardiography*, vol. 1, *The P-Q-R-S-T-U Complex* (Baltimore: Williams and Wilkins, 1951). See also Stanley Rush, "The Fiftieth Anniversary of Dr. Lepeschkin's Career," *Journal of Electrocardiography* 17 (1984): 309–12.

tree. However, Wilson became engrossed in a technical conversation, and forgot to watch the ceremony.[56]

Coda

Wilson enjoyed teaching those who were capable of following his intensive approach to the subject. He gave an annual course on electrocardiography, lecturing six to seven hours per day for five-and-a-half days. He encouraged international cooperation, especially with South America and Mexico.[57] Many of his students and colleagues became outstanding physicians and investigators.[58]

Honors started to accrue to Frank Wilson in the 1940s. The first Frank Norman Wilson Lecture in Cardiology was given at the University of Michigan on November 14, 1940, by his good friend Samuel A. Levine, on "Auscultation of the Heart."[59] Special issues of *Circulation* and the *American Heart Journal* were dedicated to him in 1950, and the American Heart Association gave him the Gold Heart Award in June, 1951.

Wilson suffered from the condition that attracted so much of his time, coronary artery disease. In 1943 he started to have precordial pain with exertion, radiating down both arms. A portable ECG machine, taken from the heart station to Wilson's Stockbridge farm, recorded a tracing that showed the presence of a myocardial infarction. Wilson suffered another myocardial infarction in Mexico City in 1946, but would not allow himself to be hospitalized and flew back to Ann Arbor in an unpressurized airplane.

In 1948 Wilson fell under a Farmhall tractor at the farm, which rolled downhill over his chest. He was noted on chest X-ray to have a pulmonary lesion, presumably tuberculosis.[60] Wilson was treated

---

56. Wilson-Lepeschkin, "Cardiologists I Have Known," 15.

57. A 1972 Mexican postage stamp features Frank Wilson. Robert A. Kyle and Marc A. Shampo, *Journal of the American Medical Association* 250 (1983): 2680.

58. A partial list of his colleagues and students is G. Canby Robinson, George R. Herrmann, Shelly Wishart, A. Garrard Macleod, Paul S. Barker, Franklin D. Johnston, Francis F. Rosenbaum, Hans Hecht, Charles E. Kossmann, Herman Erlanger, J. Marion Bryant.

59. The lecture was published in the *New England Journal of Medicine* 225 (1941): 526–32.

60. Letter from FJH [Fred Jenner Hodges] to R. H. Bayley, July 21, 1943, in Lecture Volume.

with streptomycin, at that time a very new drug.[61] The lesion failed to heal. In 1952 he was scheduled to undergo a lobectomy, but during induction of anesthesia, he suffered a cardiac arrest. He was resuscitated, but the surgery was not done.[62] Typical of his intense interest about electrocardiographic theory, at 3:30 A.M. on the morning after his cardiac arrest Wilson remarked, "You know, . . . the reciprocity theorem of Helmholtz is going to have a lot more to do with electrocardiography in the future than any of us realize."[63] Wilson returned to the farm, but died there suddenly on September 11, 1952, at the age of sixty-two.

Wilson's life and intellectual career illustrate a number of historical features about both his research project and the period in which he lived. Wilson's research differed from that of most of his medical school colleagues. Both at Michigan and elsewhere, the norm for academic medicine in the 1910s and 1920s was more empirical, clinical, or pathological research than either theoretical or instrumental work. Most researchers who focused their attention on the heart took more of a public health than a technological approach to the subject of heart disease.[64]

Wilson took a different path. During his career he strove to understand the electrical action of the heart, melding abstract theory with complex instrumentation. His theoretical studies of the QRS complex would have been impossible without both adequate empirical data and the time to contemplate its meaning. For both of these, Wilson benefited from private philanthropy, an important source of support in the interwar period. Machines such as those Wilson needed were not inexpensive, and Wilson was supported by the Horace Rackham Research Grant Program, a fund provided by a private donor who had made his fortune by filing the incorporation

61. Paul Barker to Louis Katz, September 21, 1951, in Lecture Volume.

62. Robert F. Johnston, "A Brief Account of the Scientific Contributions of Frank N. Wilson, M.D.," *University of Michigan Victor Vaughan Society Proceedings* 22 (1956–57).

63. Francis Rosenbaum, "Biography of Dr. Frank N. Wilson," handwritten document in the possession of the author, p. 5. Rosenbaum was one of Wilson's associates before moving to Milwaukee, where he enjoyed a fruitful career as a cardiologist.

64. Joel D. Howell, "Hearts and Minds: The Invention and Transformation of American Cardiology," in Russell C. Maulitz and Diana E. Long, eds., *Grand Rounds: One Hundred Years of Internal Medicine* (Philadelphia: University of Pennsylvania Press, 1988), 243–75.

papers for Ford Motor Company.[65] Apart from the cost of equipment, Wilson's theoretical bent was relatively inexpensive, requiring support for little more than his time. Once more, private philanthropy helped, though somewhat indirectly, this time by bringing Cyrus Sturgis to chair the Department of Medicine, a move that allowed Wilson and others—most notably Louis Newburgh—time to carry on their research agendas.[66] Wilson believed that research support should be given to individuals, not to projects, and that significant advances came when people had time not only for concentration but for reflection, a frequent pastime of his at the farm in Stockbridge.[67]

Wilson started his career inspired by the first generation of electrocardiographers, led by Einthoven and Lewis, and their work on arrhythmias. He soon moved to a different kind of issue, related to the study of nonarrhythmic conditions. Wilson fashioned a consistent theme throughout his career: the ventricular complex—how to measure it, how to explain its form in health, and how to interpret its variations in disease. Wilson himself explained how his work fit into the study of the ECG. He divided use of the ECG into two main rationales: to analyze arrhythmias, as Sir Thomas Lewis had done, and to study disorders of ventricular conduction, as he himself did.[68] Wilson said of the disorders first mentioned, cardiac arrhythmias, "In by far the greatest number of instances these conditions can be easily identified by inspection, palpation, or auscultation. No special knowledge of electrical phenomenon is required for their solution." This describes most of Lewis's work. It also explains why Lewis, and most English physicians, felt that the ECG was fundamentally a tool for teaching and for research, not for clinical practice.

Wilson then went on to describe his own work. "Abnormalities of the form of the ventricular complex belong in an entirely different category [from cardiac arrhythmias] . . . . They have no mechanical

---

65. Joel D. Howell, "U-M's Rackham Arthritis Research Unit," *Michigan Medicine* 88 (1989): 36–38.

66. See in this volume, "Cyrus Cressey Sturgis and American Internal Medicine, 1913–57," by Steven C. Martin, and "Louis Harry Newburgh and Metabolism at Michigan," by Steven J. Peitzman.

67. Wilson-Lepeschkin, "Three Cardiologists," 15.

68. Frank N. Wilson, Francis F. Rosenbaum, and Franklin D. Johnston, "Interpretation of the Ventricular Complex of the Electrocardiogram," *Advances in Internal Medicine* 2 (1947): 1–63.

equivalents [and] cannot be detected by any means other than an electrocardiographic examination . . . .

Then, after pointing out the unreliability of T waves as signs of myocardial disease, Wilson discussed why these two kinds of ECG abnormalities, arrhythmias and changes in the QRS, require different investigative approaches.

> Some have expressed the view that clinical electrocardiography is an empiric science . . . . Studies of this kind [measurements and statistical analyses of series of patients] are both valuable and necessary, but it is folly to assert or to imply that they are the sole road to progress in electrocardiographic diagnosis . . . . To arrive at a rational classification of abnormal ventricular complexes and to interpret them on a logical basis . . . can hardly be acquired without some knowledge of the origin of the cardiac action currents, and the principles which govern their distribution in the body.

In other words, Wilson saw medical advances as coming not from empirical clinical observation alone, but also from the application of basic scientific theory. For Wilson, that basic theory derived from mathematics and physics. In the case of the electrocardiogram, Wilson showed how basic science could lead to advances of a clinically important nature. Taken for granted in the 1990s, this is a conviction that was new and exciting when Wilson first started his studies in the 1910s.

Louis Harry Newburgh and Metabolism at Michigan

Steven J. Peitzman

Medicine in 1916

When Louis Harry Newburgh joined the Department of Medicine of the University of Michigan Medical School in 1916, American medicine and medical education were experiencing remarkable changes, some almost imperceptible, others rapid and conspicuous to those involved. Newburgh's work and career both depended upon and furthered many of the changes. As a model of a career in clinical investigation during the decades when such a thing was first possible in America, Newburgh's story may serve as a fruitful case study (fig. 12). Like all case reports, some of the findings are typical, others idiosyncratic to the subject and the setting.

What was medicine like in the period from 1910 to 1920, and what was changing? The following is a partly arbitrary selection. Although typhoid fever, tuberculosis, and pneumonia remained frequent challenges in practice, as epidemic infectious diseases declined, attention turned increasingly to the chronic and "metabolic" diseases—cancer, diabetes, hypertension, nephritis. Imported from

This work was supported by a grant from the Department of Internal Medicine of the University of Michigan Medical Center. The author is grateful to Joel Howell, M.D., Ph.D., for his help and encouragement. Courteous and skillful help was provided by the staffs of the Bentley Historical Library of the University of Michigan, and the College of Physicians of Philadelphia.

The Bentley Historical Library and the Department of Internal Medicine of the University of Michigan Medical School are both in Ann Arbor, Michigan. Copies of the Newburgh files held by the Department of Internal Medicine have been deposited in the Bentley Historical Library.

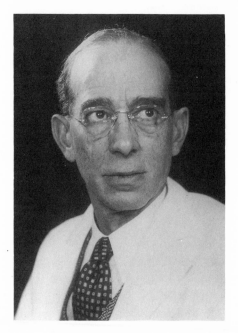

Fig. 12. Louis Harry Newburgh

Germany, the notion of "functional diagnosis" captivated many American physicians and threatened to displace pathology as the underpinning of medical science. Functional diagnosis meant using quantitative methods to determine the deficits and compensations in the workings of diseased organs; it drove the development of diagnostic laboratories and created a language of "reserve," "insufficiency," and "failure" still in use today. By 1910, most hospitals had established a diagnostic laboratory, which did mainly urinalyses, blood cell counts, and bacteriologic smears and cultures. In 1916, there existed no routine blood chemistry determinations whatsoever; blood smears and counts were made from earlobe or finger sticks, and venipuncture (done occasionally for cultures) was considered an extraordinary and invasive procedure.

But just at this time, two American workers, Otto Folin of Harvard and Donald D. Van Slyke at the Rockefeller Institute Hospital, were rapidly refining a set of analytic chemical techniques suitable for relatively rapid use with small samples of blood. Folin's colorimetric system and Van Slyke's ingenious gasometric methods allowed measurement of glucose, urea, uric acid, creatinine, total carbon dioxide, and other substances, which would enormously facilitate first investigative and eventually routine clinical work. The study of metabolic and renal disorders obviously would benefit most. Related to the growing interest in chronic and metabolic disease was a swelling interest in nutrition in the 1910s through the 1930s, a movement little discussed so far by medical historians, and about which more will be said later in this essay.[1]

Medical education underwent its own, related, changes in the first decades of the twentieth century. Lubricated (but by no means triggered) by the Flexner Report of 1910, a process gathered momentum by which marginal medical schools closed, and survivors sought to reform their educational programs. Almost universally, leaders of the better schools embraced the idea that first-rate education and research were intrinsically linked. The "full-time" system gradually took hold: schools hired qualified physicians whose tasks would be teaching and investigation, their clinical practice subservient to these primary responsibilities. Newburgh was one of many young men hired on this basis by clinical departments in the 1910s. He had the right background and the right interests.[2]

Louis Harry Newburgh's Life

Newburgh was born June 17, 1883 in Cincinnati, the son of Henry and Laura Mack Newburgh. His father succeeded in the clothing and tobacco businesses, though as a young man he had hoped to study medicine. Newburgh attended the Franklin School in Cincinnati, then Harvard College. "My social life in college was disappointing,"

---

1. There is no adequate account of the work of Folin and Van Slyke and its vast influence. Some information is available in Robert Kohler, *From Medical Chemistry to Biochemistry* (Cambridge: Cambridge University Press, 1982) and in my paper "Nephrology in America from Addis to the Artificial Kidney, in R. C. Maulitz and D. E. Long, eds., *Grand Rounds: One Hundred Years of Internal Medicine* (Philadelphia: University of Pennsylvania Press, 1988); see also the biographies of Folin and Van Slyke in Charles Gillispie, ed., *Dictionary of Scientific Biography* (New York: Scribners, 1981). The best account of "functional diagnosis" remains Knud Faber, *Nosography in Modern Internal Medicine* (New York: Paul Hoeber, 1923), 112–71.

2. For the reform of medical education, see Kohler, *Medical Chemistry*, 121–57; and for the fullest treatment, Kenneth M. Ludmerer, *Learning to Heal : The Development of American Medical Education* (New York: Basic Books, 1985).

he wrote later, for his class's fiftieth anniversary report. "This I attribute to several factors. I was unknown because I came from the middle West. I had no musical ability, nor did I possess any athletic prowess. Being very shy I made few friends." All of this changed when Newburgh began medical school at Harvard: "Life was busy and happy. In due course I became an intern at the Massachusetts General Hospital and that experience was the most thrilling of my professional career." Newburgh graduated from the Harvard Medical School in 1908.[3]

Like thousands of young American medical graduates in the period from the 1870s to World War I, Newburgh chose the scientific environment of Germanic medicine for additional training, in his case to acquire scientific methods and ideology in the laboratories and clinics of Hans Eppinger in Vienna. Eppinger's interest (stated in more or less modern terms) was the balance of sympathetic and vagal outflows and their humoral and pharmacologic relationships. On returning to the United States, Newburgh became assistant to Fred Forcheimer, a prominent physician in Cincinnati, and also started an individual practice. Unhappy with this life and wanting to "devote my best energies to medical research and teaching," he returned to Boston in 1912 as assistant visiting physician at the Massachusetts General Hospital with a junior faculty position at the Harvard Medical School. There he found the opportunity to work with important, and soon-to-be-important, figures such as biochemist Lawrence J. Henderson, and internist-investigators Walter W. Palmer and George R. Minot. Several years of work in Boston led to publications dealing with the cardiovascular response to pneumonia, cardiac output, urinary acidity in heart disease, and "the dietetic treatment of constipa-

---

3. Sources for Newburgh's life are: Obituary by James H. Means, *Trans. Assoc. Amer. Physicians* 70 (1957): 19–22; Adelia Beeuwkes and Margaret W. Johnston, "Louis Harry Newburgh—A Biographical Sketch," *J. Nutrition* 85 (1965): 3–7; materials in Newburgh files, Department of Internal Medicine, University of Michigan Medical School (hereafter referred to as UMMS), particularly copies of Harvard class reports (Class of 1905), including "Fiftieth Anniversary Report" and others not clearly identified; also in same files, typed sheet, "Information Regarding Dr. Louis Harry Newburgh, M.D.," probably prepared by his sister, Emily Newburgh Freiberg; letter, Emily Newburgh Freiberg to Margaret Woodwell Johnston, July 25, 1964. The quotations are from the Harvard class reports.

tion." This last, and least "scientific" contribution, hinted at what became a lifelong interest in dietetics.[4]

In 1916 Newburgh accepted the position of assistant professor of medicine at Michigan, with a salary of $1,600 annually. One year later, presumably to his surprise, Newburgh at the age of thirty-four found himself acting head of the Department of Internal Medicine when Nellis Foster left. In 1919 he became associate professor of medicine, and in 1922 received the unusual title, "Professor of Clinical Investigation." Except for leaves of absence during World War II, Newburgh's remaining career was spent entirely at Michigan. He retired to Southern California in 1951 and died July 17, 1956.

Newburgh married Irene Haskell of Quebec in 1912. They had two sons, Henry, born in 1915, and John David, who was born in 1920 and died in 1953.[5]

Newburgh's Research

Newburgh studied several diseases and processes concurrently over three decades. The most important of these will be reviewed thematically, not chronologically (into the 1940s, his interest in renal disease and electrolytes seems to have superseded his earlier emphasis on energy balance, obesity, and diabetes).

Classic Metabolism, Heat Exchange, and Insensible Water Loss

Nothing appeared in Newburgh's books, reviews, and lectures more frequently than this, his favorite equation:

$$\text{Insensible Loss of Weight} = H_2O + CO_2 - O_2$$

Newburgh was interested in heat exchange—the amount of heat generated metabolically and the amount discharged by the animal or person. *Why* he was interested in this will emerge later in this chapter. He wanted to estimate accurately the heat a person loses over

---

4. L. H. Newburgh, "The dietetic treatment of constipation," *Boston Med. Surg. J.* 168 (1913): 757–60.

5. Beeuwkes and Johnston, "Louis Harry Newburgh."

long periods of time. It was already known, of course, that the body loses heat by radiation, conduction, and convection, which Newburgh called the "dry method," and by evaporation, the "wet method." Each milliliter of water vaporized consumes 0.58 calories of heat, or energy. If a person goes about his or her business, normally clothed in an environment neither very hot nor cold, and avoids exertion, according to Newburgh's argument, the heat that a person loses by evaporation of the "insensible water loss" remains a relatively fixed fraction—about 24 percent—of overall heat loss. This figure varies from day to day, but is predictable when averaged over many days.

Thus heat loss can be calculated by a very careful measurement of daily "insensible weight loss," this being the difference between beginning weight and final weight, to which is added the weight of urine and feces, and from which is subtracted the weight of food and liquid ingested. But the individual also gains the weight of oxygen breathed in and loses the weight of CO_2 expelled. These weights can be estimated using the respiratory quotient so long as the subject under study is on a diet whose total quantities and proportions of fat, carbohydrate, and protein are precisely known. Newburgh placed volunteers (some paid, some his staff) and certain patients on fixed diets and had them weigh themselves, their meals, fluids, feces, and urine each day for weeks and even months in order to demonstrate the validity of this method of calculating the heat given off by the body.[6]

Nonetheless, it was challenged by others in the field of classic metabolism. To answer this criticism, Newburgh wished to compare his method, based on insensible weight change, with indirect calorimetry, an established means of measuring heat loss. To accomplish this, in April of 1934 he secured a grant from Parke-Davis Company to construct at Michigan an indirect (respiratory) calorimeter equipped with a precision balance. Newburgh spent much of 1934 setting up this complicated device, attending to the most minor details. He corresponded with Thorne Carpenter of the Nutrition Labo-

---

6. See details of this method and its justification in L. H. Newburgh and M. W. Johnston, *The Exchange of Energy between Man and the Environment* (Springfield, Ill.: Thomas, 1930), or in L. H. Newburgh, F. H. Wiley, and F. H. Lashmet, "A Method for the Determination of Heat Production over Long Periods of Time," *J. Clin. Invest.* 10 (1931): 703–21.

ratory of the Carnegie Institute of Washington.[7] The chamber contained (in addition to the balance) "a standard single bed, a chair, a table, a reading lamp, telephone and radio connection." After a series of experiments, Newburgh concluded that his insensible water method for estimating heat loss when averaged over time correlated well with the actual values obtained calorimetrically.[8]

The work and care which went into Newburgh's series of investigations of heat loss stagger the imagination: subjects on precisely prepared diets, weighing themselves and their excreta for months at a time; a unique and highly sophisticated calorimetry-balance chamber; countless Kjeldahl determinations of urine collections; an immense mass of readings and calculations. Heat loss is rarely a question in the mind of the internist of the 1990s—why did it matter to Newburgh in the 1930s? In part the results informed his theories about obesity, but to understand the context of this work, and indeed almost all of Newburgh's work, one has to know something of the history of metabolism, nutrition, and dietetics.

Digression: The History of Metabolism and Nutrition

In the later nineteenth century, the study of nutrition, as other sciences, increasingly sought quantitative methods. Knowledge concerning the utilization of protein, fat, and carbohydrate to produce energy originated in the work of Karl von Voit (1831–1908) and Max von Pettenkoffer (1818–1901), and of Voit's pupils Max Rubner (1854–1932), Wilbur Atwater (1844–1907), and Graham Lusk (1866–1932). The *calorie* was preeminent in their work, and their careers spanned and created the great age of calorimeters. The calorimeter of Voit and Pettenkofer in Munich initiated this line of diffi-

---

7. Newburgh files, UMMS: e.g., Newburgh to Carpenter, September 27, 1934; Carpenter to Newburgh, December 10, 1934. There are also letters dealing with technical requirements to Crowell Manufacturing Company of Brooklyn (blowers), Charles Foster and Warren Collins of Boston (spirometers), Troemner Balance Company of Philadelphia (modifications to balance). The grant is awarded in a letter from E. A. Sharp of Parke-Davis & Company to Newburgh, April 3, 1934.

8. L. H. Newburgh, M. W. Johnston, F. H. Wiley, J. M. Sheldon, and W. A. Murrill, "A Respiration Chamber for Use with Human Subjects," *J. Nutr.* 13 (1937): 193–201; L. H. Newburgh, M. W. Johnston, F. H. Lashmet, and J. M. Sheldon, "Further Experiences with the Measurement of Heat Production from Insensible Loss of Weight," *J. Nutr.* 13 (1937): 203–21.

cult work. With physicist E. B. Rosa, Atwater, during the years 1892 to 1896, constructed the first American calorimeter capable of studying human beings, at Wesleyan College in Connecticut. The great Sage Calorimeter at the Russell Sage Institute for Pathology in New York City produced thousands of measurements under the direction of Lusk and Eugene DuBois. As the historian Charles Rosenberg has written, "by the first decade of the twentieth century, calorimetric work had become an extremely popular, almost fashionable field, with broad implications for public policy and popular health education."

Calorimetry achieved a reductionist understanding, or at least a proud quantification, for what seemed the essence of life itself—the production of energy, the "animal heat." More practically, it provided estimates of the amount of energy consumed at rest and at work, allowing experts to recommend the amount of calories that a working man must consume in the diet to stay fit and active. This was exactly the sort of information sought by "practical" scientists and engineers of the so-called Progressive Era, roughly the period of the 1890s to World War I. One of the central themes of Progressivism was the utilization of scientific information to enhance the well-being and "efficiency" of society. But beyond this we must return to Rosenberg's hint of a fad or fashion: for those involved, there seemed to be something compelling, almost entrancing, in the production of exactly balanced numbers through calorimetric research. Newburgh's long and inexhaustible devotion to energy balance may be explained in part as scientific fashion and choice: there are trends, enthusiasms, even love affairs, in science as in life's other pursuits. The numerical crispness of balance studies, perhaps the artificer's satisfaction with the machine well built, appealed powerfully to Harry Newburgh. Newburgh included a photograph of Wilbur Atwater as the frontispiece of one of his books; he felt part of this tradition and embraced it. Newburgh was among the last of the classical calorimetrists.[9]

9. For the history of nutrition and especially calorimetry, see Graham Lusk, *Nutrition* (New York: Hafner, 1964; republication of 1933 edition in "Clio Medica" series); Newburgh and Johnston, *Exchange of Energy*, 6–26; the following articles in Charles Gillespie, ed., *Dictionary of Scientific Biography* (New York: Scribners, 1981): "Wilbur Olin Atwater," by Charles Rosenberg, 1: 325–26; "Graham Lusk," by Charles Rosenberg, 8: 555–56; "Max Rubner," by K. E. Rothschuh, 11: 585–86; "Carl von Voit," by Frederic Holmes, 14: 63–67. The quotation is from Rosenberg's article on Atwater, 325.

Related in part to advances in the understanding of normal and disordered energy expenditures, a rebirth of dietetics occurred within American and European medicine in the early twentieth century. Medical historian Fielding Garrison wrote in 1929 that "dietetics, one of the basic principles of Hippocratic therapy, has . . . come into its own again."[10] Other factors encouraging a return to diet therapy were the discovery of vitamins during the first decades of the twentieth century, and the success of liver feeding in the dreaded disease pernicious anemia.

A single library, that of the College of Physicians of Philadelphia, acquired sixty-one diet manuals in the period from 1900 to 1935; the largest number (seventeen) in any five-year period were added between 1930 and 1934. The Department of Dietetics of the University of Michigan Hospital in the mid-1920s could prepare *seventy* different diets, and such prodigious diversity was typical for larger hospitals of the period.[11] A hospital in 1930 would offer four or five ulcer diets, up to five different diets for typhoid fever, five or six for diabetes, high- and low-protein renal diets, a variety of low-salt diets, diets high or low in purine, diets to reduce constipation, others to prevent autointoxication, reduction diets and fattening diets, sometimes two or three distinct diets for arthritis, high-vitamin diets, pernicious anemia diets, ketogenic diets for epilepsy, and other assorted menus.

Not surprisingly, in the same period, dieticians saw their work sanctified by professionalization. Formal training in therapeutic dietetics began in the United States around the turn of the century, partly within nursing schools, partly within the "home economics" movement. Soon such training became available within some universities, while a few medical schools or hospitals (such as Michigan's) provided "internships" for student dieticians. The American Dietetic Association was founded in 1917, and by 1925 its educational require-

---

10. F. H. Garrison, *An Introduction to the History of Medicine*, 4th ed. (Philadelphia: Saunders, 1929), 737.

11. See James D. Bruce, "The Department of Internal Medicine," *Michigan Alumnus* 32, no. 26 (April 24, 1926). The author reviewed diet manuals in the Library of the College of Physicians of Philadelphia for Mount Sinai Hospital of Philadelphia (1934), Presbyterian Hospital of New York City (1926), and St. Mary's Hospital of Rochester, Minnesota (1932); their available number and types of diets were remarkably similar.

ments for membership included a "bachelor's degree with a major in foods and nutrition, from a recognized college or university."[12]

Thus nutrition qualified as high science through quantitative studies of metabolism, and addressed practical needs through the application of dietetic therapy in the care of the sick. Much of Newburgh's other work brought issues of nutrition and metabolism to the clinic.

Obesity

The most direct, practical product of Newburgh's calorimetry and energy-transfer studies seems to have been his conclusions about obesity. Human obesity was an increasingly recognized problem in the 1920s and 1930s, at least as judged by the appearance of articles in medical journals. Abundant controversy centered on the mechanism of fatness. Some German authorities asserted that their studies proved that the obese generate less heat from a given amount of food than the lean, even that the laws of energy conservation and transformation may not apply in this disorder.

Newburgh studied several obese subjects using his method for calculating heat production and loss over long periods of time (probably not very many subjects, since the same clinical descriptions recur in his papers and reviews—but these were not easy studies to carry out). He and collaborator Margaret Woodwell Johnston concluded that "obesity is always caused by an inflow of energy that is greater than the outflow."[13] He agreed that sometimes the clinician encountered patients who for days at a time failed to lose weight when given diets clearly below their basal metabolic caloric needs. By carefully measuring and calculating energy balance and (crucially) *water* balance in selected obese patients showing this seemingly inexplicable violation of thermodynamics, Newburgh was able to demonstrate that what actually occurred was a temporary gain of water weight. In his books and reviews he included graphs showing this phenomenon, indicating that when the water aberration is understood, the nonwater weight loss exactly follows that predicted from

---

12. See Mildred J. Chambers, "Professional Dietetic Education in the U.S.," *J. Am. Diet. Assoc.* 72 (1978): 596–99.

13. L. H. Newburgh and M. W. Johnston, "The Nature of Obesity," *J. Clin. Invest.* 8 (1930): 197–213.

energy balance. And eventually the retained water is excreted, bringing the actual weight loss into agreement with the predicted weight loss.

What then is the "cause" of obesity? It is overeating, the product of a "perverted habit." Some obese persons require "stimuli of greater intensity before they feel satisfied" (satiated). "In other persons the combination of a weak will and a pleasure seeking outlook upon life, lays the background for the condition."[14] Newburgh, as the reader might surmise, was *thin;* but these discomforting words must be heard in the setting of the 1920s and 1930s, decades not yet highly psychologized. In fairness to Newburgh, his later lectures and reviews on obesity reveal a far more sophisticated and indulgent attempt to understand overeating as an emotional response to stress and misery.[15] Newburgh treated obesity with low-calorie diets, patiently, and with a confidence built of convincing numerical data.

Diabetes Mellitus

Newburgh made two contributions to the care of persons with diabetes, both related to diet. One has endured as a cardinal observation; the other, whatever its worth, was all but eradicated by insulin.

Before insulin, the only effective treatment for what would now be termed type I diabetes was starvation or near starvation, an approach developed by Frederick M. Allen. Draconic restriction of total caloric intake did succeed in controlling hyperglycemia and ketosis, but the consequence was often cachexia and disability.[16] Newburgh found that he could keep almost all diabetics free of glycosuria and acidosis, yet provide enough energy for a reasonably normal life, by prescribing a diet in which most of the calories were obtained from fat. In 1920 he reported his success with 73 patients, and by 1922, 190 patients had been treated with the high-fat diet. Following a brief

---

14. Ibid.

15. See L. H. Newburgh and M. W. Johnston, "Obesity," *Med. Clin. North Amer.* 27 (1943): 327–47 and L. H. Newburgh, "Obesity," *Arch. Int. Med.* 70 (1942): 1033–96. (This was his most detailed review of the subject; correspondence in the Newburgh files, UMMS, shows that he received an immense number of reprint requests for this paper.)

16. See Michael Bliss, *The Discovery of Insulin* (Chicago: University of Chicago Press, 1982), especially 20–44.

period of near starvation for those patients severely out of control, Newburgh and his dieticians gradually built up the grams of fat, keeping total carbohydrate at no more than 25 to 35 grams. Protein was allowed up to about two-thirds of a gram per kilogram of body weight. The "Newburgh Four," which became legendary at Michigan, was diabetic diet number four at University Hospital; it included 220 grams of fat, 55 grams of protein, and 35 grams of carbohydrate. Patients swallowed great quantities of cream, butter, bacon, eggs, and mayonnaise.

For some years, Newburgh, who directed the care of diabetics at Michigan's hospital and clinics, had essentially all patients on this program. He did not and could not report long-term follow-up, because the introduction of insulin in the mid-1920s made both the starvation and cream-feeding of diabetics obsolete. Unless one proposes that Newburgh was either delusional or dishonest—and there is surely no reason to do so—his high-fat diet must have achieved success, at least for limited periods in many patients.[17] How this occurred metabolically remains unclear. Newburgh was not the only proponent of the high-fat diet for diabetes, and perhaps not the first; but he surely was the most fervid.

A more lasting contribution to the literature on diabetes mellitus was Newburgh's series of observations on obese, middle-aged diabetics, a group which he found were increasingly filling the diabetes clinic. He showed that, with weight reduction, most such patients lost their glucose intolerance.[18] Not satisfied with having made a useful discovery, Newburgh wished to understand what was taking place metabolically in such patients, a few of whom were induced to dwell for a time in his calorimetry chamber. His results suggested to

---

17. L. H. Newburgh and Phil L. Marsh, "The Use of a High Fat Diet in the Treatment of Diabetes Mellitus," *Arch. Int. Med.* 26 (1920): 647–62; L. H. Newburgh and Phil L. Marsh, "Further Observations on the Use of a High Fat Diet in the Treatment of Diabetes Mellitus," *Arch. Int. Med.* 31 (1923): 455–90; S. Wishart, J. Johantgen, and N. Clarke, *The Therapeutic Manual of the University of Michigan Hospital* (Ann Arbor: George Wahr, 1926). This pocket manual for pupils and house officers provides details of the high-fat diet; of interest, nearly one-quarter of its 393 pages are devoted to dietetics.

18. See L. H. Newburgh, Jerome Conn, M. W. Johnston, and E. S. Conn, "A New Interpretation of Diabetes Mellitus in Obese, Middle-Aged Persons: Recovery through Reduction of Weight," *Trans. Assoc. Amer. Physicians* 53 (1938):245–57; L. H. Newburgh, "Control of the Hyperglycemia of Obese Diabetics by Weight Reduction," *Ann. Int. Med.* 17 (1942): 935–42.

him that the obese older diabetic (the type II of present-day terminology) is better able to oxidize dietary carbohydrate than the young, lean diabetic. He therefore assumed that this group could not normally dispose of that portion of a carbohydrate load which is not promptly burned but instead forms liver glycogen. One of America's reigning authorities on diabetes, Frederick M. Allen of the Rockefeller Institute for Medical Research, never fully accepted the distinction between the two types of diabetic patients. It is difficult to be certain that Newburgh was the "first" to identify this distinction (nor does it matter very much). Certainly his combination of clinical observations with calorimetrics, and his success with weight-reduction diets, gave strong support to the argument that is now universally accepted.

Renal Disease, Water, and Electrolytes

When Newburgh was a medical student and intern in the first decade of the twentieth century, little was known about the cause of diffuse renal disease, then still termed "Bright's disease" or "nephritis." That certain acute hemorrhagic forms followed scarlet fever or tonsillitis was recognized. Exposure to cold and wetness was still thought of as an important cause of acute and chronic Bright's disease, an idea originated with Bright himself in the 1820s and 1830s.

Early in his career, Newburgh read the following statement in the 1909 edition of William Osler's popular *Principles and Practice of Medicine:*

It is quite possible that in persons who habitually eat and drink too much, the work thrown upon this organ [the kidney] is excessive, and the elaboration of certain materials is so defective that in their excretion from the general circulation they irritate the kidney.[19]

Newburgh reasoned that, "if overeating injures the kidney, the harmful effects are presumably caused by the abuse of protein, since fats and carbohydrates are broken down into carbon dioxide . . . and

---

19. Quoted in L. H. Newburgh, "The Etiology of Nephritis," *Medicine* 2 (1923): 77–104.

water," which do not require renal elimination.[20] Newburgh the nutritionist, over three decades, studied diet as irritant and later as healer of the kidney.

First, Newburgh fed a high-protein diet to rabbits, and succeeded in producing renal lesions and even symptoms suggesting uremia.[21] This initial work was published in 1919. Subsequently, with his capable collaborator Margaret Woodwell Johnston, he studied protein-rich diets in rats, and in this animal again renal lesions appeared, though of a different sort. Further refinement, however, suggested that not all types of protein-rich foods were equally able to induce renal injury. A diet made up of liver extracts was most nephrotoxic, and the effect could be reproduced by administering "sodium nucleates," that is, salts of nucleic acids.[22]

He also attempted to produce renal irritation by feeding high-protein diets to human subjects. In one experiment published in 1921, five medical students each ate one-and-one-half-pound beefsteaks at noon and at six o'clock.[23] Newburgh reported that red cells appeared in the urine of each student on the day of the study. Returning to the question some years later, he contrived to have a laboratory worker ingest a diet containing over 300 grams of protein daily for six months. This single subject showed slight albuminuria and an increase in the Addis count of cast excretion. At the conclusion of the study period, the volunteer not surprisingly became, at least for a time, a vegetarian. The casts and albuminuria vanished. Newburgh in the discussion referred to data on albuminuria among Greenland Eskimos, who habitually ingest a diet consisting largely of meat.[24]

In the 1940s, Newburgh returned once again to the relationship between diet and nephritis, now utilizing a quantitative model based on estimates of work and energy that much appealed to him. The model and concept were formulated by Thomas Addis (1881–1949) of Stanford University School of Medicine, an early authority on renal

20. Ibid, 98.

21. Ibid, 98–100.

22. L. H. Newburgh and M. W. Johnston, "High Nitrogen Diets and Renal Injury," *J. Clin. Invest.* 10 (1931): 153–60.

23. Newburgh, "Etiology of Nephritis," 102.

24. L. H. Newburgh, M. Falcon-Lesses, and M. W. Johnston, "The Nephropathic Effect in Man of a Diet High in Beef Muscle and Liver," *Am. J. Med. Sci.* 179 (1930): 305–10.

disease whose career and interests in many ways paralleled those of Newburgh. Addis reasoned as follows. An important element of the work of the kidney is to excrete urea against a concentration gradient. This work can be calculated from a formula first published in German literature in 1905:

$$\text{Work} = nRT\left(2.3 \log \frac{U}{B} - \frac{U-B}{B}\right)$$

(U and B are urine and blood concentrations of urea, or generally, solute; n is the gram molecular weight of the solute, R the gas constant, and T the absolute body temperature.)

As renal mass is lost, continued this hypothesis, remaining nephrons must expend more energy or work to sustain total urea excretion. Since overwork eventually wears out organs and tissue, rest is desirable (this was a well-established general principle of medicine for many years, particularly applicable to heart disease). Addis supported this notion with meticulous rat experiments demonstrating that animals with experimentally created renal failure showed proteinuria, sediment activity, and poor survival when given usual diets, but were protected by low-protein diets.[25] Among Newburgh's last papers were reports on the measurement of renal tubular work in man.[26] There are flaws in this line of reasoning, which relates renal work primarily to the excretion of concentrated urea. However, the relationship between dietary protein and the progression of chronic renal failure once again became a vital topic in nephrology in the 1980s and 1990s.

---

25. See Thomas Addis, *Glomerular Nephritis* (New York: MacMillan, 1948), for the full development of these ideas. For Newburgh's formulations, see L. H. Newburgh, "Renal Tubule Work: Its Significance for the Clinician," *Bull. New York Acad. Med.* 24 (1948): 137–46, and L. H. Newburgh, M. W. Johnston, and J. D. Newburgh, *Some Fundamental Principles of Metabolism* (Ann Arbor: J. W. Edwards, 1948), 45–51. J. D. Newburgh was John David, Newburgh's son, a mathematician who worked out a fuller version of the tubular work equation and calculated how renal tubular work would be changed by osmolar load: J. David Newburgh, "The Changes which Alter Renal Osmotic Work," *J. Clin. Invest.* 22 (1943): 439–46.

26. A. Camara and L. H. Newburgh, "Measurement of Renal Tubular Osmotic Work in Man," *Univ. Mich. Med. Bull.* 18 (1952): 285–96. There are, of course, flaws with these concepts of renal osmotic work, renal rest, and so forth, but space does not permit discussion of them here.

While Addis emphasized and used in his practice the low-protein diet to lessen the supposedly injurious work requirement of diseased kidneys, Newburgh (who did not refute Addis's regimen) stressed also the role of water. Water balance was another lifelong subject of Newburgh's quantitative approach to clinical issues. By ensuring adequate urine flow (water excretion) in the patient with renal disease, he felt it ought to be possible to reduce the concentration at which solutes are excreted, and thereby reduce the work required.

Newburgh, in the years after World War II, now assisted by Michigan medical graduate Alexander Leaf and grants from the Public Health Service, turned most of his attention to renal disease and related problems. Pursuing the focus on tubular function, he revived another long-time interest, the mechanism and treatment of edema. Newburgh knew that edema formation depends on salt retention, not an idea he created, but one he grasped fully. He carried the idea to an extreme, however, by doubting that water, if given alone, would be retained in edematous states. In fact, he treated many edematous patients with water loading, supposing that a more-dilute urine should favor, by gradient effects, the removal by diffusion across the tubule of "solids," such as salt. He must have induced or worsened hyponatremia in at least a few cardiac or cirrhotic patients, but this entity was not readily detected until the invention of the flame photometer around 1946; before then, measurement of plasma sodium concentration required slow and laborious gravimetric methods. His water-loading treatment for edema (which others had also proposed—it was not Newburgh's unique suggestion) was a supplement to his primary therapeutic measure, which was of course a low-salt diet. He came to understand very clearly the obligatory salt loss seen sometimes in certain nephritic patients, and knew of the danger of dietary salt restriction in such persons.

Exploring salt and water balance in more detail, Newburgh and Leaf performed some provocative studies on the handling of different salts of sodium by the kidney.[27] In this period (the late 1940s), Newburgh, Leaf, and others working with them also began studies of the control of salt excretion by adrenal hormones. Newburgh,

---

27. A. Leaf, W. Couter, and L. H. Newburgh, "Some Effects of Variation in Sodium Intake and of Different Sodium Salts in Normal Subjects," *J. Clin. Invest.* 28 (1949): 1082–90.

already into the customary retirement years, welcomed these new and "modern" ideas. Alexander Leaf left the University of Michigan in 1949. It was to Boston and the Massachusetts General Hospital, where his mentor Harry Newburgh had first acquired the passion for investigation, that Leaf returned to carry on the studies of fluid balance and renal pathophysiology that would make him a leader in this field.

Newburgh's Clinical Responsibilities

Newburgh saw private consultations, but the largest part of his clinical work was caring for inpatients and persons attending the Metabolism Clinic and the Diet Therapy Clinic. This he did, of course, with house officers and junior staff assistants. He wrote to the dean in 1936

> For several years I have been held responsible for the management of most of the diabetic inpatients and out-patients, for the nephritics and hypertensives, and a miscellaneous group of individuals presenting a variety of unusual metabolic disturbances."[28]

He added that this consumed about one-third of his time. In 1939 he reported to the chief of medicine, Cyrus Sturgis, that he had charge of "a large diabetic clinic, which consists of the in-patients. In any one day there are on the average of 50 such patients for whom we are responsible."[29] The author has not discovered any clinical case books or other materials that would provide details of Newburgh's typical "work-up" or therapy. His dietary treatments for diabetes, obesity, edema, and nephritis are implicit in his research work and publications, as already reviewed.

Two co-workers later wrote,

> Although he displayed great kindness to the patients in his care, one always sensed that even while he was at the bedside of a

---

28. Newburgh to A. C. Furstenberg, January 6, 1936, dean's records of UMMS, Bentley Historical Library.
29. Newburgh to Sturgis, July 25, 1939, Newburgh files, UMMS.

patient, he was impatient to hurry back to the laboratory to determine the basis for the chemical phenomena operative in the disease under study."[30]

Newburgh as Teacher

Newburgh enjoyed protection of time for his research, but taught medical students and dieticians in the wards and classrooms. Although his assignments varied during his more than thirty years at Michigan, probably typical was the academic year 1938–39. He made "teaching ward rounds" three mornings a week for two months, and "gave a half-hour clinic" weekly. This latter activity was probably an informal discussion of a selected outpatient under care for a disease of special interest to Newburgh. He also taught a ten-hour lecture course for junior students on nutrition, and judging by the number of letters in various files relating to its scheduling and length, no doubt Newburgh cherished his hours in the proprietary tradition of medical school faculty members. A list of the lecture topics for 1936–37 shows that the "Junior Lectures in Nutrition" amounted to a series of talks on Newburgh's favorite research themes, with almost nothing about vitamins and little on nutritional deficiencies. Here again, one readily detects a durable and exasperating custom of medical education.[31]

Newburgh almost surely was at his best when teaching on the wards with small groups of students, correlating the patient's complaints and symptoms with the available information from the laboratory. He was superbly capable of offering sophisticated and lively metabolic and pathophysiological interpretations.

Newburgh, the Man

Available letters written by Newburgh deal mostly with professional matters and reveal little personality. As this essay is being prepared, in the early 1990s, many persons are still alive who knew and worked with him in his later years, and who could undoubtedly flesh out this

---

30. Beeuwkes and Johnston, "Louis Harry Newburgh," 6.

31. This section is based on "Administrative Information Sheet," "Faculty Instruction Record," and related notes; typewritten "Topics—Junior Lectures in Nutrition, 1936–1937," all in the Newburgh files, UMMS.

portrait. This writer has inferred the following from written sources and from the recollections of several persons who knew Newburgh. He was a serious-minded person who, it is just to conclude, did not suffer fools gladly. He was probably not outgoing or effusive. He surely gained the lasting respect and affection of many colleagues and friends. But, often single-minded in his scientific opinions, he could be dogmatic. Two long-time co-workers admitted that his "loyalties and convictions sometimes led to controversy, which at times unfortunately became bitter."[32]

Outside of his work, his life centered on his family and home, to which he was devoted. As it does eventually for every man or woman, time mixed grief with joy in Newburgh's family life. His brilliant son David died in 1953, a few years before Newburgh himself. Ironically, Mrs. Newburgh possibly suffered with a disease her husband no doubt counted as one of the curiosities of his clinics, adrenal insufficiency. She remained reasonably well, however, once adrenal extract was secured. With his wife, Harry Newburgh shared a love of gardening, and their home and terraces became a beautiful showplace. The Newburghs seemed to enjoy conventional vacation trips to Canada or other destinations. Beyond this, Newburgh had no particular hobbies or avocations.

He was not an outwardly religious individual, nor does he seem to have been politically active. In response to a Harvard class survey of 1935, when asked his opinion of the New Deal, Newburgh—ever the nutritionist—replied, "baloney." Surprisingly, in another class report from 1946 he is listed as "socialist."[33] Science, medicine, family, and home (no order of priorities is intended) seemed to fully engage his mind and energy.

Newburgh and the University of Michigan Medical School

Newburgh's career at Michigan spanned thirty-five years. He retired in the spring of 1951, the occasion ceremonially marked on June 18 by an enthusiastically attended dinner and the presentation of a

---

32. Beeuwkes and Johnston, "Louis Harry Newburgh," 7.
33. Copies of class reports and records, Harvard College Class of 1905, in Newburgh files, UMMS.

handsome engraved wristwatch. What was the meaning, or value, of Michigan to Newburgh, and of Newburgh to the university, especially its Department of Medicine? What elements fostered such a long and fruitful alliance? What does his career tell us about internal medicine and clinical investigation during their formative decades in the United States?

First, what did Michigan mean to Newburgh? As a young physician he felt a thirst for research and the generation of new knowledge. His ambitions clarified just at a time when American medical schools decided to embrace research and build faculties of teacher-investigators. Michigan provided a suitable, though not perfect, matrix for his aspirations. Laboratory space was made available. A modest salary (which most full-time clinical faculty could supplement with limited patient fees) abolished the need to practice for a living. What few, if any, schools provided, however, was adequate financial support for work in the laboratory. Probably few deans or boards of trustees recognized that investigation required the hiring of fellows, technicians, and the purchase of rats, dogs, and all manner of equipment.

Newburgh's long career demonstrates the transition from private support of research to governmental sponsorship. Although many similar investigators in American medical schools won support from patients, friends, and local philanthropy, Newburgh was especially fortunate in his setting. After relying on help from his own family for some years, his research program secured a $20,000 grant in 1928 from the Fellowship Foundation of Battle Creek (this was, of course, money from Kellogg's Corn Flakes). No doubt the Kellogg people saw Newburgh's work in nutrition and metabolism as a highly compatible object of philanthropy. Later, he obtained substantial funding from the Horace H. Rackham and Mary A. Rackham Fund. This fund, derived in part from family holdings in the Ford Motor Company, has been a major source of support for the University of Michigan. His later work in renal tubular function and electrolyte metabolism won a grant from the Public Health Service (equivalent to an NIH grant) in 1947.[34]

---

34. For information on Newburgh's grants (there were others not mentioned in text), see: Reports of Regents, University of Michigan, 1923 to 1949 (indexed references under "Newburgh"); also a typed summary of references to Newburgh in these Regents' Reports, found in the dean's records, UMMS, box 53, Bentley Historical Library;

Most important, Newburgh's time was protected. It was understood that he was appointed in large part to carry out investigations. This is the basis for his unusual title, as of 1922, professor of clinical investigation. Only a few schools ever awarded this title, or the similar "professor of medical research," and an occasional school set up a separate department of medical research or research medicine (for example, the University of Pennsylvania). These may be thought of as transitional, or tentative arrangements, in a period when a few faculty members in a school were considered the designated researchers. The next stage, arrived at by most medical schools, yet still a perplexing assumption, would be the expectation that *everyone* on the full-time faculty be an investigator. But for Newburgh the title surely helped defend his time to do research. For reasons obscured by the years, Louis Warfield, who served briefly as chairman of the Department of Medicine, attempted in 1924 to assign morning clinic hours to Newburgh, under the supervision of a more-junior faculty member. The dean, Hugh Cabot, reversed this action, agreeing that it amounted to "interference with their work" (Newburgh's collaborator Philip Marsh was to have manned the afternoon clinic).[35] Never again would Newburgh find unreasonable educational or administrative obstacles standing in the way of his research.

The medical school setting also provided patients, the substrate for much of Newburgh's most-important work. Again a particular event illustrates this function. In 1938, Newburgh requested authority to "manage all diabetic patients on the medical service." Although it must have been no simple affair, in a memorandum of September 28, 1938, the chairman of medicine, Cyrus Sturgis, agreed to the request. Newburgh would have permission at least to see every diabetic admitted, and "any of the cases which he sees could be desig-

---

correspondence, proposals, statements of research purposes relating to Newburgh in Horace A. Rackham and Mary A. Rackham Fund Papers, box 15, Bentley Historical Library; correspondence concerning United States Public Health Service grant RG 743 to Newburgh, in dean's records, UMMS, box 50, Newburgh files, Bentley Historical Library; Marjorie Cahn Brazer, *Biography of an Endowment* (Ann Arbor: Rackham Board of Governors, 1985).

35. Cabot to Warfield, September 30, 1924, dean's record, UMMS, Bentley Historical Library.

nated by him for special study . . . . [T]he purpose of this is to facilitate teaching and research in diabetes."[36]

Obviously, the medical school environment also supplied capable house officers and students to look after much of the clinical workload, allowing the professor of clinical investigation more time for his experimental work. Some of these would see the attraction of Newburgh's metabolic studies and become his fellows or pupils. The increasingly common presence of collaborating basic scientists in the clinical departments of a medical school, such as Newburgh's close associate Margaret Woodwell Johnston at Michigan, represents another facilitating factor. But Newburgh does not seem to have collaborated often with investigators in the "basic science" departments. Clearly, a strong medical school such as Michigan's could attract bright students and residents, sick patients, and wealthy friends; all of these contributed to Newburgh's forging a successful career in clinical investigation.

Finally, what was the meaning of Newburgh's life to the University of Michigan Medical School? Certainly, it was not found in the acquisition of research grants, which in Newburgh's day were necessary for his work but did not bolster the Medical School, as NIH grants would come to do later. After a while, Newburgh's cumulative scientific knowledge and bedside experience must have made him a valuable teacher on the hospital floors, but not an indispensable one. Rather, Newburgh's immense value to the Medical School, especially during his early years, was what his work said about the school and how it wished to be seen.

When "full-time" and the ideology of research came to departments of medicine in the 1910s and 1920s, internal medicine as a scientific pursuit was categorized in many schools (not always "officially") into three divisions: metabolism, cardiology (especially electrocardiography), and microbial diseases. Newburgh's choice—metabolism—comprised classical heat and energy measurements, nutrition, and indeed almost any investigation of disease that utilized quantitative chemical measurement. Renal disease, gout, diabetes, obesity, electrolyte disorders—all fell into the category of "metabolism." Newburgh's classical metabolic investigations brought science

---

36. "Memorandum in Reference to the Request of Dr. Newburgh to Manage All Diabetic Patients on the Medical Service," September 28, 1938, with addendum, October 4, 1938, Newburgh files, UMMS.

in its most quantitative, rigorous form, to medical research—brought the techniques of physics and chemistry to study the very hallmarks of life, heat and energy, in the sick and the well. In the 1920s and 1930s, there was no more pure and serious form of science housed in a medical school clinical department than that carried out by Harry Newburgh.

At the same time, the study of metabolism, through its virtual identity with the study of dietetics, attended to a most practical yet sanctified question of the clinic: choosing a regimen, selecting the feeding that would restore the sick person to health. In the 1920s and 1930s, physicians, including academic physicians, looked to diet as a major element in the treatment of internal disease. Indeed, in those days before the advent of hypertrophied technology, a sick person came to hospital in good part for its special milieu: freedom from the normal efforts of life, rest, nursing, and a prescribed diet.

So, as Louis Harry Newburgh's name acquired national and even international fame through his presentations, lectures, and publications (in the best American medical journals), his presence at the University of Michigan Medical School made several statements. These statements were: high science is conducted there and new methods of treating the sick are discovered there. These are the ways in which a medical school wanted to see itself, when Harry Newburgh tested his dietary ideas with his beloved balance-calorimeter, and how a medical school wants to be seen today.

L. H. Newburgh: A Remembrance

Alexander Leaf

My acquaintance with L. H. Newburgh determined my career in medicine. The acquaintance began in my first year of medical school at the University of Michigan and was purely fortuitous. Dr. Newburgh had a son, David, who was also starting medical school in the same class with me, in 1940. David was brilliant, the closest I have come to knowing an intellectual genius. I was drawn to David, and we soon became close friends. Dr. Newburgh noted our friendship and assumed erroneously that any friend of David's must also be exceptionally gifted. So I got adopted into the family and, therefore, had many opportunities to meet with Dr. Newburgh informally at his home, as well as to see him less frequently in the hospital later during my clinical rotations.

Most unfortunately, David became ill with ulcerative colitis during our first year and had to drop out of medical school. He had a stormy course with his illness but, for a time, was sufficiently in remission to obtain a Ph.D. in mathematics, in which subject he also exhibited great promise. While he was a junior faculty member several years later, after I had finished medical school, David had a severe recurrence of his colitis and died.

I mentioned this tragic occurrence because of its effect on Dr. Newburgh. He was immensely and appropriately proud of David and, as is often the case with fathers of brilliant offspring, his own happiness was tied to David's accomplishments. David's death was an exceptionally tragic event in Dr. Newburgh's life, one from which he never fully recovered during his last years. Dr. and Mrs. Newburgh had one other child, a son a few years older than David, who was an engineer of superior intelligence, but apparently not in David's class.

Dr. Newburgh had an inquiring mind and was always curious about all scientific matters. His field of special interest was energy metabolism, a field in which he was certainly outstanding. He made many meticulous measurements of human energy production, having built a whole-body calorimeter in which precise measurements of oxygen consumption and carbon dioxide production could be made on a subject or patient, who was incarcerated within the chamber for days or weeks. Dr. Newburgh made notable contributions to our understanding of obesity from such painstaking studies. He demonstrated that the failure of many obese individuals to lose weight promptly while on a low-calorie diet and in negative calorie balance was not due to a failure of human metabolism to adhere to the second law of thermodynamics as claimed by a German authority, but rather to simple water retention. By continuing his observations and measurements of caloric balance for a longer period than did his German colleague, and following insensible water losses by a method he had devised, he noted a brisk diuresis and his subject's weight would fall exactly to that expected from the negative caloric and fluid balance.

Dr. Newburgh was a firm believer in the dictum that science begins when quantitative measurements are made. Much of medicine in his day was simple clinical and pathologic description, and he was one to usher in the era of experimental medicine and insisted on careful quantitation of all biologic parameters. He was highly regarded for the rigor of his measurements in energy, fluid, and electrolyte metabolism, in which fields he was an internationally recognized authority. But son David chuckled as he described how his father, after reading of Einstein's studies on gravity and relativity, had placed balances in the basement and the top floor of University Hospital and weighed his patients at both levels to see whether their weights would be less on the top floor than in the basement of the hospital!

When David was ill, I spent many weekend afternoons at the Newburghs' home and listened with fascination while the professor talked about his research interests or some other subject close to his heart. It was an unusual opportunity for a young medical student to have such a close personal relationship with a distinguished senior professor. He often talked while we both weeded his garden, as he and Mrs. Newburgh were ardent horticulturists. Often he grumbled about the quality of education, both medical and nonmedical. He was most enthusiastic about the increasing application of science to medicine, but he decried and was very disappointed by medical students' lack of science training.

His esteemed medical peers were individuals like Dr. Eugene DuBois at the Russell Sage Institute in New York, whose metabolic chamber served as a prototype for his; Drs. John P. Peters of Yale and D. D. Van Slyke, of the Rockefeller Institute, whose pioneering measurements of body fluids and electrolytes he admired; Dr. Thomas Addis, the Stanford nephrologist, who had introduced quantitative methods into the evaluation of kidney diseases; and Dr. James Gamble, the Harvard pediatrician, whose studies of fluid and electrolyte metabolism in humans had opened a new field. These were a few of the leaders in medicine at that time, and all were close friends of Dr. Newburgh's. Each spring, with the arrival of the clinical meetings, which in those days were held in Atlantic City and were the major annual academic meetings in medicine, Dr. Newburgh got increasingly excited as he looked forward to discussing his research results and interests with these colleagues and others.

When I finished medical school, Dr. Newburgh urged me to have my internship in Boston. He was always proud of his medical school days there and often spoke of his experiences as a medical resident and junior faculty member before he came to Michigan. In those days, there were many formalities in Boston medicine. Dr. Newburgh described how Dr. Frederick C. Shattuck, the Jackson Professor of Clinical Medicine at Harvard and chief of medicine at the Massachusetts General Hospital, arrived at the hospital for rounds in morning dress. The house staff were at the entrance to meet his arrival. The door was held open by the lowly interns, and the residents were lined up according to rank on either side as Dr. Shattuck swept into the Bulfinch Building.

In those days, medicine was practiced according to authoritative precepts. Dr. Shattuck had devised his own regimen for the treatment of typhoid fever, namely to starve the patients, allowing them only fluids. Dr. Newburgh, then an intern, had a young mother on his ward who had typhoid fever and was receiving the Shattuck therapy. He watched her become progressively weaker while she pleaded for food. Finally, as a gesture of kindness one evening Dr. Newburgh seeing her gradually slipping away, brought her steak and potatoes, which she devoured. The next morning on rounds, Dr.

Shattuck noted the striking improvement in the young woman and demonstrated to his coterie of attentive residents the success of the Shattuck regimen. When he was informed that the patient had been fed a hearty meal the night before, he was furious and called Dr. Newburgh to his office, where he scolded him for his disobedience and threatened him with expulsion. So much for experimental medicine under authoritarianism, concluded the young Dr. Newburgh.

I didn't see much of the Newburghs while I was in Boston, though the family rented a cabin in Duxbury for the summers. One weekend, I was invited to spend a couple of days with them. Dr. Newburgh was working for a National Research Council project on naval research at that time. One of the serious problems was with pilots shot down over the North Sea and Atlantic, who parachuted into the ocean and survived less than an hour in the frigid waters. Dr. Newburgh had designed a light suit that the aviators could wear over their clothes. The material was alleged to permit evaporation of sweat to avoid overheating while working but at the same time to provide a waterproof, thermal protection from the freezing waters.

I learned that one reason for my invitation to Duxbury was to test the new suit. Since the project was classified, the testing had to be done very secretly. About midnight, Dr. Newburgh helped me don the suit and I waded into Duxbury Bay. I hardly got in up to my middle before it was all too apparent that the suit was leaking like a sieve. I'm not sure they ever designed a suit with the properties they were seeking, but many of our most senior faculty were busy traveling back and forth to Washington to help with the war effort.

On discharge from military service, I returned to the University of Michigan at Dr. Newburgh's invitation to serve as an instructor in medicine and to do research in his laboratory. Upon my arrival, Dr. Newburgh was most cordial and helpful. He had a newly assigned laboratory space in the basement of University Hospital where he took me and told me that this was my laboratory. He offered to help me with whatever needs I had, but there was one stipulation. I was never to come to him asking what I should be doing. If he knew the answer to that, he said, I wouldn't be there, as he would be doing the research himself. It was a wonderful time for me. I started some balance studies to determine how the body regulates its sodium content. I was joined by a medical resident and medical student, and we did our metabolic studies on each other. There were, of course, many discussions with Dr. Newburgh, which all of us enjoyed.

We often discussed how one starts a research project. He expressed a view I don't share, but which in those days seemed attractive. He thought it was sufficient just to start making measurements of humans with whatever analytical procedure one had confidence in, and soon a legitimate project would make its appearance from the resulting numbers. To support his view, he would cite the great German physiologist, Max Rubner, whom he said always started his projects in that manner. I suppose in those early days of this century, there was such a dearth of quantitative data that collecting measurements of any biological parameter soon led one to specific questions to investigate. Needless to say, such an approach is not likely to win an NIH research award today.

Dr. Newburgh was meticulous in the quality of the laboratory data he sought, and he urged us to be similarly thorough in our analyses. I remember when we showed him a discrepancy in the measured sodium intake of our subject and the measured loss of sodium in urine and stools; he suggested that we measure the sodium losses from the skin. This entailed washing down our naked subject with distilled water, while collecting the washings in a sodium-free basin in which he stood, and keeping him unclothed for twenty-four-hour periods on sheets that had been pre-rinsed with distilled water. At the end of each twenty-four-hour period, the subject was again rinsed with distilled water, the washings combined with the rinse water from the sheets, and analyzed for sodium content—about 22 to 75 mgs per day for nonsweating subjects, I recall—a painfully tedious process.

Often in our discussions, Dr. Newburgh would say, "You can ask me how the body does something, but never ask me 'Why?' That question you should address to God." Dr. Newburgh was not a religious person in the conventional sense, but he was filled with reverence and wonder about Nature.

Dr. Newburgh was always alert to new laboratory methods, and one day he saw in *Science* a new method for measuring sodium and potassium, called flame photometry. Analysis for these two most-important biological ions was incredibly tedious and, in fact, I was convinced required a small measure of voodoo, as well. We were both excited by this new method, and he brought back from one of his trips to New York a couple of selenium barrier-type photocells, light filters, a galvanometer, and a Meaker burner. With a bit of local glass blowing and wires, I put together one of the first flame photometers.

Having the instrument assembled, I asked my laboratory technician for half a dozen urine specimens that she had analyzed. At that time, we were doing balance studies on a nephrotic patient whom we kept on a very low-salt intake. The sodium concentration in the patient's urine was less than 1.0 mM, and it took my excellent technician about one week for each urine determination. With my crude flame photometer, I ran off the six urine specimens for sodium and potassium in about thirty minutes. When I compared the flame photometer results with those obtained laboriously by my technician, the agreement was excellent. My technician was crestfallen, and the next day she resigned; her redundancy was staring her in the face!

The time finally arrived when our first studies were completed and I could write them up for publication. Dr. Newburgh insisted that I have this experience myself. He made me use clear, concise English with impeccable grammar. It was a real struggle for me, but the happy day came when he was satisfied with my prose. When I brought him the final manuscript, I had included him as a coauthor. He objected to this and insisted that I remove his name. I was initially depressed by this, thinking that he felt the paper was not up to the quality with which he wanted his name to be associated, but that was not his point. He said the ideas and work were mine, and he wanted to be certain that I received full credit for the research.

When I protested that he had certainly been most helpful and supportive and that without him the studies would never have been done, he indicated a recent paper in the *Journal of Clinical Investigation* in which we had been very interested that came from Thomas Addis's laboratory at Stanford. Dr. Addis's name appeared on that paper as the last author. Dr. Newburgh told me that if I could name the first author on that paper, he would let me put his name on my paper. We had been referring to the paper as Addis's study and, needless to say, he had made his point. Such generosity by established investigators to their younger colleagues is unusual today, but the lesson was one I have never forgotten.

That time spent with Dr. Newburgh was among the happiest of

my academic career, but things were not so comfortable at home. By then, I had acquired a wonderful wife, and our first daughter was then a little over one year old. My support was to be the $110 per month coming from my veteran's benefits, to which Dr. Newburgh agreed to add another $100 from his research funds. My wife and I knew things would be tight even in those days on this stipend, but she knew what I wanted and never made even a murmur of complaint. We would have managed on this, and Dr. Newburgh's share came regularly monthly, but the expected check from the Veterans Administration just didn't arrive. After several months of this, and with my wife losing weight and our infant perpetually chilly in the drafty cabin during the frigid winter, I went to Dr. Newburgh to complain that we couldn't continue in that way. He told me he would see what he could do about the matter, but first he gave me a little lecture, saying that that is what *they* do to individuals who want to go into medical research. His own path had not been made easy. Eventually, and happily, the checks from the Veterans Administration began to arrive.

There was austerity in the laboratory as well. We had to be frugal with all reagents, even with paper and writing materials. Nothing that was reusable was ever discarded. Whenever possible, we fashioned our own equipment. We had firsthand knowledge of every procedure done in the laboratory and were comfortable using and, when necessary, repairing all the equipment. Equipment was much simpler then, but one didn't get misled by some software package that was inappropriate for the task at hand. This all took place just before the NIH began to subsidize medical research in 1948 and before the explosions occurred in molecular biology. Though things were simpler in those days, I have always cherished the privilege I had in being introduced to medical research under Dr. Newburgh's benevolent, wise, and personal tutelage.

Thomas Francis, Jr.: From the Bench to the Field

Naomi Rogers

Medicine in America 1900–1928

In 1928, Thomas Francis, Jr. a promising young scientist, went to New York City to work at the Rockefeller Institute for Medical Research. His study of the immunology of respiratory diseases was promising, and he could have stayed in this mainstream track of clinical and virological investigation. But by the mid-1930s, Francis had begun to reject both these traditions—as a researcher at the bench or by the bedside—for work in the field as an epidemiologist. His work in the 1940s and 1950s on influenza and polio, epidemic diseases of significant public health concern, helped to establish epidemiology as a major field of medical research, and himself as a leader in his profession (fig. 13). In 1953 he was chosen to design and evaluate trials of the Salk polio vaccine, a massive task that brought him international attention and acclaim.

Despite his achievements in virology and epidemiology, Francis is largely forgotten today by physicians and historians. His efforts to transform medical research and education by incorporating what he termed the "epidemiological approach" was until recently overlooked and ignored. Scientific medicine of the early twentieth century, histo-

The research for this work was supported by the Department of Internal Medicine of the University of Michigan Medical School. For their comments and critiques of this work, I would like to thank Maureen Dyer, Hughes Evans, June Factor, Joel Howell, Susan Lederer, John Harley Warner, members of the Alabama History of Medicine and Science Group, and the two anonymous readers for the University of Michigan Press. Various people have shared their memories of Francis with me; my thanks in particular to Frederick Epstein, Mrs. H. Davenport, James Neel, Nicholas H. Steneck and Myron Wegman.

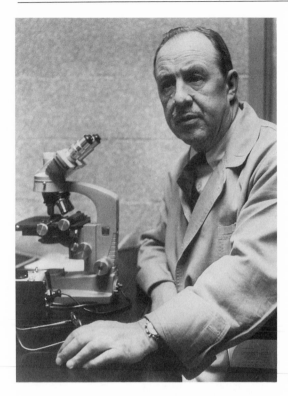

Fig. 13. Thomas
Francis, Jr.

rians have argued, provided a narrow and confining direction for
American medical professionals. But Francis attempted to continue a
tradition of environmentalism and preventive medicine, refusing to
be bounded by research oriented only to the laboratory or the bedside. In the 1950s he told an international conference on medical
education that "Epidemiology extends the boundaries of the universe
in which the disease can be viewed well beyond the ward or clinic.
It provides a third dimension to the understanding of disease by
creating awareness of the nature of the environment in which the
disability arises."[1] In his efforts to work within this "third dimension"
Francis helped to push American medical research beyond the bench
and the individual patient to the community.

Francis (1900–1969) was born in Gas City, Indiana. His father, a
steelworker and a Wesleyan Methodist lay preacher, had immigrated

---

1. Thomas Francis, Jr., "The Teaching of Epidemiology," *Proceedings: First World
Conference on Medical Education* (London: Oxford University Press, 1953), 635.

with his family from Wales to the United States just before Francis was born.[2] In 1921, after graduating with a bachelor of science degree from Allegheny College in Meadsville, Pennsylvania, Francis chose to study medicine at Yale University. His choice of Yale was influenced by Yale's new professional prominence. In 1917, while Francis was at high school in Newcastle, Pennsylvania, Yale had hired a new dean, Milton C. Winternitz, a student of the eminent Johns Hopkins pathologist, William H. Welch. Winternitz began to redesign Yale's medical school based on the Johns Hopkins model of employing prominent researchers and teachers full time, including an impressive group of investigators in internal medicine.[3]

Francis's early interest in the study of respiratory disease was kindled by his experience, while at college, as a member of the Student Army Training Corps during the 1918 influenza pandemic. "I remember how the sick men looked and behaved," he later wrote. Influenza, he reflected, "was truly a lethal biological bomb and medicine could only stand by, pathetically helpless, to observe and record and speculate."[4] His experience in the 1920s at Yale, as a medical student, an intern, a resident at New Haven Hospital, and an instructor in internal medicine, reinforced his interest in clinical research as a way to improve doctors' skills at the bedside. "It became apparent," he later commented, "that there was little to offer in the way of treatment" for many diseases; doctors needed "new knowledge" about "the nature of the microorganisms and viruses—whence they came, how they behaved, and how they could be countered. The atmosphere in which I was working was enticing and so without previous planning I turned to research on disease."[5]

The medical world that Francis entered was challenging and swiftly changing. With the rise of scientific medicine in the 1880s and 1890s, the laboratory had become the new but contested locus of

---

2. John R. Paul, "Thomas Francis, Jr., July 15, 1900–October 1, 1969," *Biographical Memoirs* (Washington, D.C.: National Academy of Sciences, 1974), 44: 57–58 (hereafter referred to as Paul, "Francis, Jr.").

3. Paul, "Francis, Jr.," 58–60, and John R. Paul, "Thomas Francis, Jr., MD, as a Clinician, 1900–1969," *Archives of Environmental Health* 21 (1970): 247–48 (hereafter referred to as Paul, "Clinician"). Francis also chose Yale influenced by the experience of his physician brother-in-law, who trained there.

4. Thomas Francis, Jr., "Adventures in Preventive Medicine," *Allegheny College Bulletin* 3 (1959): 10.

5. Francis, "Adventures in Preventive Medicine," 10.

medical research and discovery, as two main traditions of medicine—clinical practice and laboratory work—struggled to become "scientific." The impressive successes of bacteriology and immunology reinforced the belief of many physicians that research at the laboratory bench was more promising for improving patient care and professional status than clinical work. But ambitious academic clinicians sought to transform their field by integrating the new scientific methods at the hospital bedside. What these approaches had in common was a narrowing of the research focus and a rejection of medical research in the community at large.

Epidemiology in this period seemed far from the scientific cutting edge. Distant from a laboratory or a bedside, the methods of epidemiology were associated with an older tradition of medicine: sanitary science and its theoretical basis, the filth theory of disease. Sanitary science had developed in the nineteenth century as part of a broader reform movement in which physicians and other health reformers sought to improve urban society by cleaning up water, food, and the streets. The link between sanitary science and the investigation of disease was reinforced by the epidemiological work of investigators such as John Snow and William Budd in their insightful studies of the spread of cholera and typhoid. By the turn of the century, however, proponents of a new public health movement attacked sanitary science as antagonistic to the germ theory and to scientific medicine. Filth, they argued, was a vague, old-fashioned explanation of the cause and transmission of disease, and the proper direction of medical research should be to identify and explore the nature of the distinct etiological agents of disease through the bacteriological methods developed by Louis Pasteur and Robert Koch. In the 1890s Charles V. Chapin, a fervent promoter of the germ theory and new scientific medicine, placed the laboratory at the center of his public health work in Providence, Rhode Island, and urged other health officials to do the same.[6]

Scientific medicine at the turn of the century did not just promote a different kind of research; the laboratory had a larger symbolic importance. A focus on germs and laboratory techniques, medical reformers hoped, would loosen the tie between medicine and politics.

---

6. See James H. Cassedy, *Charles V. Chapin and the Public Health Movement* (Cambridge: Harvard University Press, 1962).

In the nineteenth century, American public health boards were part of urban party machines; doctors often practiced without state licenses or formal qualifications; medical societies and licensing boards were bitterly divided by political and sectarian conflicts; and medical schools varied substantially in standards. The emphasis on making American medicine scientific was part of broader reform efforts by American physicians to raise their professional status and to take control of the definition of medical standards and care away from local and state politicians. As doctors sought to appeal to the public as experts in the management of epidemics, childbirth, child rearing, and mental illness, professional medical reformers claimed science as a tool for objective investigation as well as increased prestige.[7]

By the early twentieth century, reliance on laboratory research to improve health and to cure disease seemed highly promising. Bacteriologic and immunologic techniques could, for example, effectively control the dreaded children's disease diphtheria with the use of diphtheria antitoxin. But experience with a number of other diseases threatened to undermine this optimism. At the same time, despite Chapin's New Public Health movement, physicians confronted the limited power of the laboratory in the lay community. Despite an effective treatment and a diagnostic test for syphilis, for example, the public stigma of the disease discouraged physicians from reporting cases and patients from admitting their infection. Tuberculosis was also stigmatized, and both patients and doctors similarly resisted public health guidelines. Further, despite sanitary reform of sewage, drinking water, and milk, cases of typhoid continued to flare up.[8] And some members of the public fervently resisted official efforts to put the New Public Health into practice. New York City

---

7. Paul Starr, *The Social Transformation of American Medicine* (New York: Basic Books, 1982); John Harley Warner, "Ideals of Science and Their Discontents in Late Nineteenth-Century America," *Isis* 82 (1991): 454–78.

8. Of the many useful studies of venereal disease and tuberculosis in the Progressive Era, see Allan M. Brandt, *No Magic Bullet: A Social History of Venereal Disease in the United States since 1880* (New York: Oxford University Press, 1985); Daniel M. Fox, "Social Policy and City Politics: Tuberculosis Reporting in New York, 1889–1900," *Bulletin of the History of Medicine* 49 (1975): 169–75; Michael E. Teller, *The Tuberculosis Movement: A Public Health Campaign in the Progressive Era* (Westport: Greenwood Press, 1988); Georgiana Danielle Feldberg, "'An Antitoxin of Self Respect': North American Debates over Vaccination against Tuberculosis, 1890–1960," Ph.D. thesis, Harvard University, 1989; Richard A. Meckel, *Save the Babies: American Public Health Reform and the Prevention of Infant Mortality, 1850–1929* (Baltimore: Johns Hopkins University Press,

officials' arrest of the Irish immigrant woman known as Typhoid Mary raised thorny issues of civil liberties. The resistance by German and Polish immigrant communities to compulsory smallpox vaccination and the continuing influence of antivaccination and antivivisection groups demonstrated that integrating the new sciences into medicine had not resolved ethnic and cultural tensions.[9]

The example of influenza was particularly devastating both to the American public and the medical profession. The influenza pandemic of 1918–19 caused mass hysteria. More American soldiers died of influenza and its complications than of combat injuries, and its spread in the civilian population was just as horrific. Health officials and members of the military recognized the importance of controlling this disease. But before the 1930s, laboratory research did not provide convincing ways to deal with influenza. Its etiology remained unclear. In 1899 Richard Pfeiffer had drawn attention to what he argued was the bacterial agent of the disease, but his idea remained controversial. In 1931 Richard E. Shope, an animal pathologist at the Rockefeller Institute's Princeton laboratories, identified an influenza virus in swine and claimed it was related to the human pandemic of 1918.[10] But professional and intellectual tensions between bacteriologists and virologists meant that Shope's work was greeted initially with skepticism. Many bacteriologists distrusted the work of those involved in creating the new discipline of virology, particularly when its tenets (such as that viruses required living cells for multiplication) seemed to contradict some of the basic postulates of bacteriology founder Robert Koch.[11]

1990); and Barbara Bates, *Bargaining for Life: A Social History of Tuberculosis, 1876–1938* (Philadelphia: University of Pennsylvania Press, 1992).

9. Judith Walzer Leavitt, *The Healthiest City: Milwaukee and the Politics of Health Reform* (Princeton: Princeton University Press, 1982); see also Judith Walzer Leavitt, "'Typhoid Mary' Strikes Back: Bacteriological Theory and Practice in Early Twentieth-Century Public Health," *Isis* 83 (1992): 608–29.

10. Harry F. Dowling, *Fighting Infection* (Cambridge: Harvard University Press, 1977), 195–202. See also Alfred W. Crosby, *America's Forgotten Pandemic: The Influenza of 1918* (Cambridge: Cambridge University Press, 1989 [1978]).

11. See Greer Williams, *Virus Hunters* (New York: Alfred S. Knopf, 1960), 214–15; A. P. Waterson and Lise Wilkinson, *An Introduction to the History of Virology* (Cambridge: Cambridge University Press, 1978); Sally Smith Hughes, *The Virus: A History of the Concept* (New York: Science History Publications, 1977). On the concern to "satisfy Koch's postulates for bacterial diseases," even in influenza research, see Thomas Francis, Jr., "The Immunology of Epidemic Influenza," *American Journal of Hygiene* 28 (1938): 66.

epidemics would later lead to the development of an influenza vaccine and the concept of the multiantigen viral vaccine.[24] With these research achievements, Francis could have confidently looked ahead to a career as an academic clinician and virological investigator. But, as John R. Paul, a Yale epidemiologist and medical historian, later commented, "Influenza being the kind of disease that it is, and with the 1918 pandemic fresh in almost everyone's mind, Dr. Francis was pitched forcibly into the field of epidemiology."[25]

As Francis's interest in epidemic influenza led him to explore the disease's appearance in the population, he began to publish articles on the epidemiology of influenza. Because of his background in clinical medicine and his training at the Rockefeller Institute in laboratory virology, Francis did not see epidemiology in its standard form as the study of epidemic disease, with the role of the epidemiologist to discover the cause, source, and means of transmission of inexplicable outbreaks. Rather, clinical epidemiology, as Francis and other promoters began to term it, was an activist discipline, requiring the integration of laboratory, clinical, and field research.[26] Epidemiologists, he argued, should not see themselves as subordinate to laboratory or clinical diagnosticians. They "should bring to bear the investigative power of laboratory procedures and apply them to the problem at the community level . . . . Epidemiological investigation must use whatever can be employed to detect and explain rather than to describe and leave the rest for others to interpret."[27] Under this rubric, the field could encompass the study not only of epidemic diseases but also more complex problems such as explicating the role of German measles in pregnant women, predicting and preventing serum hepatitis, and even tracing noninfectious associations, such as cigarette smoking and lung cancer.

During the 1920s and 1930s, the new discipline of epidemiology

Francis, Influenza, and American Virology, 1928–41

When Francis first began his research career in the late 1920s, virology represented the growing chasm between laboratory research and clinical practice. Despite its promise to help physicians fight frightening epidemics, virology seemed largely abstract, a concern of scientists around a laboratory bench. Virologists searched for biological properties based on mostly negative evidence, involving a search for an element not retained by bacterial filters, usually not visible in a microscope, and not grown on artificial media.[12]

In 1928 Francis, a young clinical investigator, entered the heady world of virological debate at the Rockefeller Institute for Medical Research in New York City. The institute, established by industrialist and philanthropist John D. Rockefeller in 1903, was intended to demonstrate an American commitment to medical research based on the German model of enabling scientists to work without teaching responsibilities.[13] During the 1920s and 1930s, virology became one of the most exciting areas of medical research, an era known later as the Golden Age of Virology.[14] Concepts of the nature of viruses were swiftly changing, both theoretically and through advances in radioactive tracing, chemical analysis, and later electron microscopy. In 1928 a new generation headed by Thomas Rivers, who identified themselves as virologists rather than bacteriologists, published the collection *Filterable Viruses*, arguing that viruses were distinct from bacteria, and that their study required specialized skills and knowledge.[15]

Despite the insights of scientists during the interwar years, not until the 1940s and 1950s did virology in the United States successfully achieve discipline unity.[16] There were few private institutes

24. Francis, "Recent Advances in the Study of Influenza," 251–54; Thomas Francis, Jr., "Epidemiological Studies in Influenza," *American Journal of Public Health* 27 (1937): 211–25.

25. Paul, "Francis, Jr.," 68.

26. Thomas Francis, Jr., "Epidemic Influenza: Studies in Clinical Epidemiology," *Annals of Internal Medicine* 13 (1939): 915–22.

27. Thomas Francis, Jr., "What Is the Place of the Epidemiological Approach in Medical Science?" Symposium on the Epidemiologic Approach to the Problem of Pregnancy Wastage, Arden House, New York, March 23–25, 1958, box 58, Francis papers, Bentley Library, 6–7.

12. Hughes, *Virus*, 97–98, 104.

13. George Corner, *A History of the Rockefeller Institute 1901–1953: Origins and Growth* (New York City: Rockefeller Institute Press, 1964), 24–28, 150–58; Naomi Rogers, *Dirt and Disease: Polio before FDR* (New Brunswick: Rutgers University Press, 1992), 21–22.

14. [Unknown], "Banquet Address: 37 Years On," 10, [1969], box 89, Francis papers, Bentley Historical Library, University of Michigan, Ann Arbor (hereafter referred to as Bentley Library).

15. Thomas M. Rivers, ed., *Filterable Viruses* (Baltimore: Williams and Wilkins Co., 1928); Saul Benison, ed., *Tom Rivers: Reflections on a Life in Medicine and Science* (Cambridge: MIT Press, 1967); and Paul, "Clinician," 249.

16. Paul, "Clinician," 249.

where scientists could work full time on research. Nor did researchers agree on the structure of viruses or even the nature of viral diseases. Even at the prestigious Rockefeller Institute, a center for viral research, there were major disagreements over the nature of viruses. In the 1910s and 1920s, Simon Flexner, an eminent pathologist and head of the institute's laboratories, refused, for example, to integrate his laboratory research on polio with the work of clinicians at the institute's hospital who were equally interested in the disease. Flexner was committed to animal experimentation as the way to understand the nature of both viruses and germs, and played down the gastrointestinal symptoms clinicians had noted among polio patients and other aspects of polio's distinctive epidemiology. Flexner's lack of interest in polio's epidemiological and clinical picture helped to reinforce his theory of polio as a disease spread by droplet infection and primarily affecting the nervous system, mistaken ideas that twisted the direction of polio research for at least two decades.[17] In contrast, Francis, by temperament and training, consistently sought to integrate laboratory experimentation and clinical investigation into his research.

Research work on influenza initially went slowly. As late as the 1930s, scientists were not certain that it was a viral disease, and debated how to identify the infected and the immune. Outbreaks of influenza in the 1920s and 1930s further exacerbated fears of another pandemic. In 1933, a critical date for all future studies of the disease, Christopher Andrewes, Patrick Laidlaw, and Wilson Smith at the National Institute for Medical Research in London isolated the first human influenza virus, later known as Type A. Within a few years, Smith managed to grow the influenza virus in chick embryos, and George K. Hirst, a New York pathologist, developed a simple diagnostic blood test for the disease.[18] With the identification of the etiol-

ogy of influenza and a simple way to diagnose the infected, many doctors hoped that effective control was a straightforward next step.

Francis was the first American researcher to take advantage of the London virologists' work. Indeed, a colleague later commented "his life and work encompassed the period when most of our present knowledge of influenza was developed."[19] Initially, Francis had worked at the institute's hospital in the pneumonia service as a clinical investigator, pursuing research he had begun at Yale under Francis G. Blake.[20] His interest from the outset concerned the applicability of etiologic insight to clinical practice. In the early 1930s, he and his Rockefeller colleagues published a series of studies on the serological reactions of pneumonia products as ways to measure the infective process. Francis also continued his private clinical work and established important social and professional connections, including among his private patients in New York members of the Rockefeller family.[21]

By the mid-1930s Francis had established himself as a promising virologist. In 1934 he published his first important virology study, "Transmission of Influenza by a Filterable Virus," in *Science*, the first American scientist to confirm the London virologists' isolation of the influenza virus. In 1936 Francis and his colleague Thomas Magill established antigenic differences in the virus, and in 1940 were the first to isolate a distinct new viral strain of influenza, later known as Type B, documenting that there were different types of influenza viruses and leading to the demonstration of antigenic variations in influenza.[22] In 1936 Francis moved to the Rockefeller Foundation's International Health Division, where he worked mainly on the immunology of influenza.[23] His efforts to explain the complexity of antigenic variation of the influenza virus and the role of this variation in

---

17. See John R. Paul, *A History of Poliomyelitis* (New Haven: Yale University Press, 1971); Rogers, *Dirt and Disease*; Saul Benison, "Poliomyelitis and the Rockefeller Institute: Social Effects and Institutional Response," *Journal of the History of Medicine and Allied Sciences* 29 (1974): 74–93; Saul Benison, "The History of Polio Research in the United States: Appraisal and Lessons," in Gerald Holton, ed., *The Twentieth Century Sciences: Studies in the Biography of Ideas* (New York: W. W. Norton, 1972), 308–43; and Saul Benison, "Speculation and Experimentation in Early Poliomyelitis Research," *Clio Medica* 10 (1975): 1–22.

18. Thomas Francis, Jr., "Recent Advances in the Study of Influenza," *JAMA* 105 (1935): 251–54.

19. Hershel E. Griffin, "Thomas Francis, Jr., MD: Epidemiologist to the Military," *Archives of Environmental Health* 21 (1970): 252–255.

20. Paul, "Clinician," 249; Paul, "Francis, Jr.," 60–64.

21. Paul, "Clinician," 249–50; Paul, "Francis, Jr.," 63.

22. Thomas Francis, Jr., "Transmission of Influenza by a Filterable Virus" *Science* 80 (1934): 457–59; Thomas Francis, Jr., "A New Type of Virus from Epidemic Influenza," *Science* 90 (1940): 405–408; T. P. Magill and T. Francis, "Antigenic Differences in Strains of Human Influenza Virus," *Proc. Soc. Exp. Biol. Med.* 35 (1936): 463–66; Charles H. Stuart-Harris, "Control of Influenza: Lack of Knowledge versus Lack of Application of Knowledge," *Archives of Environmental Health* 21 (1970): 276–85.

23. Francis struggled for respect against the better-known work of the Rockefeller "yellow fever boys," see [unknown], "Banquet Address: 37 Years Onward," 6.

became increasingly separated from its nineteenth-century and Progressive Era sanitary reform roots, but its proponents continued to promote what was now termed preventive medicine. The professional importance of this approach was exemplified by the opening of the Johns Hopkins School of Public Health and Hygiene in 1919 and by the work of epidemiologists in the U.S. Public Health Service such as Wade Frost, who later became a teacher and professional leader at the Hopkins school.[28] Interest in broad preventive measures against disease in this period reflected widespread concern over the large number of draftees in poor physical condition, reported after the Great War, and also medical and popular skepticism about the safety of vaccines against viral diseases. This skepticism was reinforced by the disastrous failure of experimental polio vaccines tested in New York City and Philadelphia in the 1930s.[29]

The fascinating but problematic antigenic shifts of the influenza virus meant that a vaccine developed from the viral strains currently identified might not protect against a new strain. The influenza antigenic shift, Francis reminded his colleagues, "is not limited in importance to a mere academic demonstration but adds enormously to the difficulties of eradication of the agent and seriously complicates the problems of specific prophylaxis and therapy."[30] Thus, Francis's work on viral disease reinforced his feeling that prevention was the most effective way of controlling disease, and that this concept must be integrated into American medical research programs. After all, he later wrote, "no longer could one conceive of medicine as the practice of waiting for someone to get sick and then try with our still feeble efforts to cure him. There are no cures for virus disease."[31]

Francis's professional positions in New York did not reflect this movement toward epidemiological research and preventive medicine: he held the chair of bacteriology at New York University's College of Medicine from 1938 until 1941, with visiting positions at New

---

28. See Elizabeth Fee, *Disease and Discovery: A History of the Johns Hopkins School of Public Health and Hygiene, 1916–1939* (Baltimore: Johns Hopkins University Press, 1987); and Kenneth F. Maxcy, ed., *Papers of Wade Hampton Frost: A Contribution to Epidemiological Method* (New York: Commonwealth Fund, 1941).

29. John R. Wilson, *Margin of Safety* (New York: Doubleday, 1963), 47–58; Rogers, *Dirt and Disease.*

30. Francis, "Immunology of Epidemic Influenza," 72.

31. Francis, "Adventures," 10.

York's Bellevue and Willard Parker hospitals.[32] But his influenza work pushed him beyond the traditional concepts and methods of laboratory research and clinical investigation. In 1941, as he prepared to leave New York for a new field and new position reflecting his new research interests, he told his former dean that, "It is with definite regret that I make this decision and I am doing it entirely because I think the new position offers an opportunity for the broad epidemiological scope which seems to be my trend."[33] Throughout his life, his strong training in clinical investigation and bench virology continued to influence his efforts to integrate epidemiology into mainstream American medical research.

Francis and the Military, 1941–60

World War II altered the direction of American medicine and science and reinforced many of Francis's new interests. In 1941 Francis was offered two important new positions that changed both his life and the direction of American epidemiology. Henry F. Vaughan, dean of the University of Michigan's new School of Public Health, offered him the chair of the school's epidemiology department. Although leaving the professional and social advantages of New York City was difficult, Francis sought the independence of his own research unit. One of his colleagues later commented, "he wanted his own show and he wanted the best possible show."[34] And by the 1950s Francis had established Michigan as a great center of research in virology and epidemiology. In the same year that Francis moved to Ann Arbor, he was asked by Francis G. Blake, his former teacher at Yale and now president of the Armed Forces Epidemiological Board, to head the board's newly organized Commission on Influenza. The commission was made up of a group of consultants, including epidemiologists, clinicians, pathologists, bacteriologists, and virologists. The military asked this group to develop civilian teams to help control any outbreaks of disease among the unprecedented numbers of American

---

32. Paul, "Francis, Jr.," 70. This position was still called "bacteriology" in this period, reflecting the incomplete disciplinary success of virology.

33. Francis to Currier McEwen [Dean of the New York University College of Medicine], April 9, 1941, box 2, Francis papers, Bentley Library.

34. [Unknown], "Banquet Address: 37 Years Onward," 7.

troops.[35] In his role as military consultant, Francis was able to turn Michigan into a center for military research on respiratory disease and for the training of army medical personnel.[36]

World War II was a turning point for American medicine. The structure of medical training and practice developed during the war offered many local physicians their first introduction to Big Medicine and its technological and biological products. Through the Committee on Medical Research, the federal government became the major source of funding for scientific research, and contracts were continued after the war, first through the Public Health Service and then through the National Science Foundation, established in 1950. The impressive military support of medical research during the 1940s led to the widespread use of numerous important medical innovations such as penicillin and the blood bank.[37]

By the 1940s the idea of organizing the diagnosis and prevention of disease on a large scale had gained significant military attention in spite of the still-limited professional interest in epidemiology. With the memory of the influenza pandemic of the Great War, and after dealing with a serious outbreak of influenza in 1940 that affected more than 19,000 American soldiers, American military commanders turned to civilian physicians for measures to prevent and control disease.[38] In 1941 the Army established the Board for the Investigation and Control of Influenza and Other Epidemic Diseases, later known as the Epidemiological Board. In addition to supporting

35. Griffin, "Epidemiologist," 252–55; Fred M. Davenport, Edwin H. Lennette, and Gordon N. Meiklejohn, "Origins and Development of the Commission on Influenza," *Archives of Environmental Health* 21 (1970): 267–72; Thomas Francis, Jr., "Influenza," in Ebbe Curtis Hoff, ed., *Preventive Medicine in World War II* (Washington, D.C.: Office of the Surgeon General, 1958), 4: 114–16.

36. The military commented on his relative "naivete" concerning military organization, but also his "mental alertness, scientific curiosity, and penchant for action," Griffin, "Epidemiologist," 255.

37. Joel D. Howell, "The Invention and Development of American Internal Medicine," *Journal of General Internal Medicine* 4 (1989):127–33.

38. On the history of epidemiology, see Franklin H. Top, ed., *The History of American Epidemiology* (St. Louis: C. V. Mosby Co., 1952); John R. Paul, *An Account of the American Epidemiological Society: A Retrospect of Some Fifty Years* (New Haven: Yale Journal of Biology and Medicine, Academic Press, 1973); Abraham M. Lilienthal, ed., *Times, Places and Persons: Aspects of the History of Epidemiology* (Baltimore: Johns Hopkins University Press, 1980); and Naomi Rogers, "Dirt, Flies and Immigrants: Explaining the Epidemiology of Poliomyelitis," *Journal of the History of Medicine and Allied Sciences* 44 (1989): 486–505.

bacteriological research and the development of biological products, the board coordinated mass immunological testing using the methods and skills of epidemiology.[39]

During the war, Francis worked both as an epidemiologist and as an administrator with broad powers and responsibilities. He developed and tested an influenza vaccine for America's largest wartime army, improving methods for virus purification and preparation. These disease control measures were closely watched and imitated by federal and state public health bodies.[40] Like other civilian researchers, Francis found that the military wanted medicine that worked and that was also safe and easy to administer. The Armed Forces Epidemiological Board asked Francis to develop a killed-virus vaccine against influenza, fearing that a vaccine using a live virus incompletely attenuated might infect rather than protect soldiers.[41]

During the 1940s, Francis turned the University of Michigan student body as well as parts of the Army corps into a massive pool of experimental subjects. In fact, in an aside, Francis later compared epidemiology to a scientific laboratory. Epidemiology, he commented in 1958, "represents in essence the use of the scientific method in the study of disorders concerning population groups generally. (Basically, the same as a laboratory experiment ... it is experimental)."[42] Francis's design of the influenza vaccine trials included strict controls for both patient and doctor, using double-blind and placebo methods, and later served as a model for his design of the Salk polio vaccine trials. He and his team improved the technical methods of preparing massive amounts of influenza vaccine and the logistics of administering and testing a vaccine on a large scale. In recognition of this work, Francis later received numerous professional awards, including the Medal of Freedom and the American Public Health Association's Lasker Award. He was elected a member of the National Academy of Sciences in 1948.[43] Francis's work in the military left him a lifelong supporter of killed-virus vaccines.

---

39. Francis, "Influenza," 114–15.

40. Davenport et al., "Origins and Development," 270–74; Paul, "Francis, Jr.," 72–73.

41. Francis, "Influenza," 117–18.

42. Francis, "What is the Place of the Epidemiological Approach?" 7–8.

43. Other awards included the Ricketts Award from the University of Chicago (1952) and membership in the American Academy of Arts and Sciences (1960).

The success of Francis's influenza-vaccine trials was undermined, however, by continuing influenza epidemics after the war. An influenza epidemic in 1947 with a significant antigenic shift that left vaccinated soldiers unprotected indicated the need for international attention to epidemic influenza, and for methods of including new strains into vaccines swiftly and effectively. "Dr. Francis considered this experience a milestone in the progress of knowledge rather than a vaccine failure," one of his Michigan colleagues later commented.[44] After the war, the United States was not chosen as the leading center for international funding of influenza research. In 1948 the World Health Organization based its newly organized World Influenza Center in London under virologist Christopher Andrewes. Andrewes established a system of international watch laboratories and continued the development of multivariant vaccines. As the United States became less central for cutting-edge influenza work, and American physicians more confident in their ability to control the disease through new multivariant vaccines, Francis's interests after the war shifted to other areas.

Francis's experience in the military forced him to define and defend his evolving concept of epidemiology and its place in medical and public health work. As well as dealing with respiratory-disease prevention, his work involved troop housing problems, cases of serum jaundice and hepatitis, and the use of penicillin.[45] This work reinforced his evolving view of epidemiological possibilities going beyond the identification and control of epidemic disease outbreaks.

Whether working with the military or with civilians, Francis faced professional and political resistance to his evolving concept of epidemiology. Although a Republican Party supporter and a strong believer in hierarchical direction, Francis's view of medicine grew increasingly progressive, particularly in the context of the narrowing boundaries of the American medical profession's vision of its social role and responsibilities.[46]

Francis sought to transform the concerns of physicians beyond individual patient care to preventive medicine, often quoting Rockefeller executive Alan Gregg's dictum, "Practice does not make per-

44. Davenport et. al., "Origins and Development," 271.
45. Griffin, "Epidemiologist," 253–54.
46. [Unknown], "Banquet Address: 37 Years On," 8.

fect."[47] His efforts, however, were made difficult by the organized profession's lack of interest in public health concerns, and the low status of preventive medicine in the profession; many physicians, he commented, regarded preventive medicine as "largely a field of missionaries and zealots."[48] This attitude can be seen in satirist Sinclair Lewis's influential 1925 novel *Arrowsmith*. Lewis caricatured public health activism through the figure of Almus Pickerbaugh, a midwestern public health booster. In contrast, Lewis's protagonist, bacteriologist Martin Arrowsmith, after dabbling ineffectively in public health work, finally embraced what Lewis portrayed as the purity and apolitical nature of true science: laboratory research.[49]

At the Army Training School that Francis had helped establish at the University of Michigan, he faced similar views among clinicians whom the Army sought to turn into epidemiologists. In 1943 Francis complained to Kenneth Maxcy, a Hopkins epidemiologist, that the men in "our Army group . . . have offered the comment that they thought too much Statistics and Sanitation were being given. This strikes me, however, as being the normal response of any group of men who have been essentially limited to practice."[50] Francis began to develop a series of lectures and articles criticizing what he saw as the narrow training and vision of medical education that was oriented solely to clinical and laboratory investigation. In 1949 he told a meeting of the American Medical Association, under the title "The Family Doctor: An Epidemiological Concept," that the modern physician "can advance as a conservator of health and in the promotion of preventive medicine."[51] A few years later, he invited "the clinician and the diagnostic laboratory worker to extend their horizons rather

---

47. See, for example, Thomas Francis, Jr., "The Expanding Role of Epidemiology in Medical Research," 1, March 27, 1958, box 53, Francis papers, Bentley Library.

48. Francis to William S. Tillet [New York University College of Medicine], February 21, 1953, box 7, Francis papers, Bentley Library.

49. Sinclair Lewis, *Arrowsmith* (1925; reprint New York: New American Library, 1961); Naomi Rogers, "Germs with Legs: Flies, Disease and the New Public Health," *Bulletin of the History of Medicine* 63 (1989): 599–617; and Charles E. Rosenberg, "Martin Arrowsmith: The Scientist as Hero" in Charles E. Rosenberg, ed., *No Other Gods: On Science and American Social Thought* (Baltimore: Johns Hopkins University Press, 1976): 123–31.

50. Francis to Kenneth Maxcy [Johns Hopkins], February 2, 1943, box 2, Francis papers, Bentley Library.

51. Thomas Francis, Jr., "The Family Doctor: An Epidemiologic Concept," *JAMA* 141 (1949): 311.

than restrict them," by rejecting the "great tendency" to "create a cleavage" between the fields of epidemiology and clinical medicine.[52]

Many American physicians found their military experience changed their professional life. Francis was no exception. His experience as Influenza Commission advisor and troubleshooter, and the professional connections he made during the war, helped him become a leader in epidemiology and viral research in the postwar medical world. Elements of Francis's military work continued after 1945. He remained head of the Influenza Commission until 1955, and an active member of the Armed Forces Epidemiological Board until 1960.[53] As American politicians and the military began to fight the cold war, the board's mission expanded beyond monitoring the health of military personnel to monitoring the health of the American public at large. Its members discussed "epidemiologic intelligence" and how to deal with the United States population under emergency conditions such as a nuclear attack.[54] During this period, Francis's reputation as a leading epidemiologist also grew, and he became a consultant to the Michigan State Department of Health, the American Cancer Society, and the Communicable Disease Center. These positions reflected the broadening of epidemiology beyond an emergency response to a concern with the problems of noninfectious and endemic diseases.

One of the most significant outcomes of Francis's military experiences was his involvement in the Atomic Bomb Casualty Commission (ABCC) organized by the U.S. National Academy of Sciences. The commission was established immediately after the war to deal with the scientific and social ramifications of the atomic bomb explosions, and to study the delayed effects of radiation on survivors in Japan. By the early 1950s, there were some serious problems in the project's mission and structure, partly as a result of its efforts to organize a corps of American and Japanese physicians, statisticians, nurses, technicians, interpreters, and field workers, as well as to work within

---

52. Thomas Francis, Jr., "Correlations in Clinical and Epidemiological Investigation," *American Journal of Medical Sciences* 226 (1953): 376. This was a speech he gave in 1952 to the New York State Association of Public Health Laboratories.

53. Griffin, "Epidemiologist," 254–55. Francis was president of the board from 1958 to 1960.

54. See correspondence, 1955–60, Armed Forces Epidemiological Board, box 53, Francis papers, Bentley Library.

Japanese patterns of health care and win the goodwill and cooperation of survivors. There was also a growing sense of frustration that
the initial study was providing few scientific results for researchers
under continuing stress that was exacerbated by the Korean conflict
and spiraling Japanese inflation.

In 1955 Francis was asked by the National Academy to head a
committee to visit Japan and review the prospects and objectives of
the ABCC and to propose possibilities for the future. His committee
redefined the commission's objectives and strategies, and suggested
a way of establishing a fixed population for research based partly on
the model of Francis's Army vaccine trials. Francis's team also proposed a comparative analysis of mortality, regular examinations of
exposed and unexposed cases, and short-term, intensive studies of
special diseases.[55] The efforts by his committee and by the ABCC to
transform survivors into research subjects and at the same time demonstrate concern for their health was a delicate and complex task, and
the topic remains an important one for further historical study.

Francis at Michigan, 1941–69

In 1941 medical training at the University of Michigan was trans-
formed with the founding of a separate new School of Public Health
funded by the Rockefeller and Kellogg Foundations.[56] The School of
Public Health became rooted in Michigan's medical world and grew
under the leadership of Dean Henry Frieze Vaughan. One of the
strengths of the early years of the school was its department of epidemiology, today the only remaining department of the original three.[57]
Francis, described as "perhaps the most eminent member of the faculty" in the postwar period, headed the department for twenty-eight
years, and established it as a major research and teaching center.[58]

---

55. R. Keith Cannan, "Contribution to the Work of the Atomic Bomb Casualty
Commission (ABCC)," *Archives of Environmental Health* 21 (1970): 263–66.

56. Henry F. Vaughan, "The School of Public Health," in Walter A. Donnelly,
ed., *The University of Michigan: An Encyclopedic Survey* (Ann Arbor: University of Michigan Press, 1958), 4: 1527–34.

57. The original three were public health practice, epidemiology, and environmental health, Vaughan, "School of Public Health," 1528.

58. Myron E. Wegman, "School of Public Health," in Ferol Brinkman, ed., *The
University of Michigan: An Encyclopedic Survey*, (Ann Arbor: University of Michigan
Bentley Historical Library, 1977), 5: 258.

The highlight of his work at Michigan, at least judged in terms of international media attention, came in 1955 with his announcement of the results of the Salk polio vaccine trials that he had designed and directed at Michigan. This work established a place for Michigan in American medical history. Dean Vaughan later described it as "the greatest mass experiment in the field of medicine ever undertaken."[59]

When historians look back at Francis's career today, his polio work often overshadows his other achievements. In fact, in 1955, he complained that "I have become a little sensitive that some people seem to think that the Francis Report was the only thing I ever did."[60] Yet, to a large extent, his polio work was the culmination of his medical and military experiences up to that point.

By the 1940s, polio epidemics had become a major medical and public health problem, growing in strength and frequency, and with doctors unable to prevent, predict, or cure the disease. Polio as an epidemic disease had become visible only in the early years of this century. At first it was believed to resemble the character of other epidemic diseases, associated with immigrant children in urban slums. But victims such as Franklin Delano Roosevelt helped to transform its popular image into a danger for all Americans, irrespective of class or ethnicity.[61] In 1937 President Roosevelt founded the National Foundation for Infantile Paralysis, which become one of the largest and most powerful private medical funding agencies in the 1930s and 1940s. American virologists and epidemiologists engaged in polio research also benefited from improvements in techniques for serological diagnosis and for laboratory cultivation of viruses. This work shifted the view of polio from primarily a disease of the central nervous system to a general systemic viral infection centered in the intestines. By the late 1940s, scientists concluded that polio's appearance in epidemic form, once every two or three years, was due to the infection of previously unexposed groups and the existence of more than one type of polio virus.[62]

After he arrived at Michigan, Francis began his first concerted investigations of polio, influenced in part by a theory that polio was spread like a respiratory disease, and certainly by the ready availabil-

---

59. Vaughan, "School of Public Health," 1532.
60. Quoted in Williams, *Virus Hunters*, 212.
61. See Rogers, *Dirt and Disease*, 165–75.
62. See Paul, *History of Polio*, and Rogers, *Dirt and Disease*.

ity of substantial research funds from the National Foundation for Infantile Paralysis.[63] He brought to Michigan a liberal grant from the National Foundation, which provided funds not only for research on polio and other viral diseases, but also for the training of young investigators.[64] One promising young virologist was Jonas Salk. Francis had first met Salk in 1939 at New York University, and they had worked together on efforts to kill the influenza virus with ultraviolet radiation. In 1942 Francis helped Salk get a National Foundation fellowship to come and work at Michigan. Salk stayed for almost six years, and, during the war, also through Francis's influence, joined the Commission on Influenza. Salk worked mainly on the army influenza vaccine trials with Francis, and as his major assistant developed administrative polish, technical virtuosity, and a philosophical grasp of viral diseases. In 1947 Salk left Ann Arbor for Pittsburgh to head his own laboratory; there, funded partly by the National Foundation, he developed a killed-virus vaccine for polio.[65]

In 1953 the National Foundation decided to test and promote Salk's new vaccine. It was made clear by federal research agents and prominent American virologists that the trials needed to be designed and run by someone eminent enough in the scientific world to be considered independent of politics and partisanship. The National Foundation itself was under some suspicion by conservative members of the science community for its uncritical self-promotion of so-called polio "cures" it had funded.[66]

---

63. During the early 1940s, Francis published studies of polio's relation to tonsillectomies and to the housefly, and he continued his studies of polio's serological epidemiology.

64. See Vaughan, "School of Public Health," 1532; and see Kenneth Maxcy [Johns Hopkins] to Francis, February 15, 1944, box 2, Francis papers, Bentley Library. See also Peter A. J. Cusack to Henry Vaughan [University of Michigan School of Public Health], June 21, 1944, box 6, School of Public Health, Bentley Library. Francis also received grants from the Armed Forces for research on influenza and other respiratory diseases. Between May 1940 and May 1943, Michigan received $230 thousand from the National Foundation; see "National Foundation News Release," May 20, 1943, box 6, School of Public Health, Bentley Library.

65. Richard Carter, *Breakthrough: The Saga of Jonas Salk* (New York: Trident Press, 1966), 32–36. On Salk's work, Carter, *Breakthrough*, 42–47, and Paul, *History of Polio*, 414–19; Jonas Salk, "The Restive Spirit of Thomas Francis, Jr. Still Lives," *Archives of Environmental Health* 21 (1970): 273–75. See also Jane S. Smith, *Patenting the Sun: Polio and the Salk Vaccine* (New York: William Morrow & Co., 1990).

66. Myron E. Wegman, "Francis—An Appreciation," *Archives of Environmental Health* 21 (1970): 231, quoting Carter, *Breakthrough*. Carter also wrote that "Francis's

Francis was asked to direct the Salk polio vaccine trials, a task one of his colleagues later described as "titanic and crucial."[67] Why he was chosen is a complex question. He had established himself as a scientist of integrity, an efficient, no-nonsense man who shared Salk's faith in killed-virus vaccines.[68] Francis was respected in many fields, represented by his participation in professional societies including clinical investigation, virology, and epidemiology.[69] His influenza research had raised immunological problems similar to those of polio, and left him aware of the importance of viral variation in developing a vaccine. Francis had worked for a number of years with public and private funding agencies, but he was not their slave, and could resist any media hype, thereby retaining the respect of his conservative scientist colleagues, something Salk in the late 1950s was sadly unable to do.

Unable to control the trial volunteers as strictly as he had in Army days, Francis turned to the school system as his organizing structure. Through the Polio Vaccine Evaluation Center that he established at the University of Michigan, he designed and conducted the field trials of the Salk vaccine, the largest-ever clinical study using human subjects, involving finally some 1.8 million American children at fifteen thousand schools in forty-four states. Francis had to battle with the Vaccine Advisory Committee of the National Foundation, which had already proposed vaccinating second-grade child volunteers in areas with a high incidence of the disease, and comparing

---

independence had to be conspicuous and authentic." See also Allan M. Brandt, "Polio, Politics, Publicity, and Duplicity: Ethical Aspects in the Development of the Salk Vaccine," *International Journal of Health Services* 8 (1978): 257–70; and Aaron E. Klein, *Trial by Fury: The Polio Vaccine Controversy* (New York: Charles Scribner's Sons, 1972).

67. Myron E. Wegman, "Thomas Francis, Jr.—An Appreciation," 3, ms, 1970, box 89, Francis papers, Bentley Library; Paul, *History of Polio*, 426–32. Francis may also have felt an obligation to the National Foundation after it had contributed to the building of Michigan's School of Public Health, despite the Foundation's policy against "bricks and mortar" funding; Carter, *Breakthrough*, 227–28.

68. See Francis to Luther Terry [Surgeon General], September 29, 1962, box 11, Francis papers, Bentley Library, and Alexander Langmuir [Chief, Epidemiology Branch, Communicable Disease Center] to Francis, December 3, 1962, box 11, Francis papers, Bentley Library.

69. In 1945–46, Francis was president of the American Society of Clinical Investigation; in 1947, president of the Society of American Bacteriologists; in 1949–50, president of the American Association of Immunologists; in 1951, chair of the Epidemiology section of the American Public Health Association; and in 1954–55, president of the American Epidemiological Society.

them to nonvaccinated groups of first- and third-grade children. Francis, however, felt relying on observation as the only control was not scientific enough; he saw this less as a clinical trial than as a mass epidemiological experiment.[70] He insisted on an additional double-blind placebo study involving first-, second-, and third-grade children, which Salk later attacked, calling it a "fetish of orthodoxy."[71] Commentators described the design as "pure Francis," particularly his fervent resistance to outside publicity during the year-long assessment process, and his independence from the National Foundation.[72] In particular, Francis's use of placebos showed his attitude to the reliability of evidence from ordinary clinicians. In 1954 he told the American Academy of Pediatrics that scientific research must go beyond the "limited and uncontrolled observations by some one who thought his patients responded better [with a new drug] than usual."[73]

On April 12, 1955, at the University of Michigan's Rackham Auditorium, Francis announced that Salk's vaccine was safe, potent, and effective. The announcement was a mass media event and a great success for Francis, Salk, the National Foundation, and the University of Michigan. Within a few years, however, American health officials had rejected the Salk vaccine for an oral vaccine based on an attenuated virus, developed by Salk's scientific competitor Albert Sabin.[74] Sabin's vaccine is now the major vaccine against polio used by American public health agencies. Francis, however, never accepted the higher risks involved in Sabin's use of live rather than

---

70. In 1957 Francis described the polio vaccine trials as "great epidemiological experiments." Thomas Francis, Jr., "Epidemiology and the Future of Medicine," June 10, 1957, *University of Tennessee Record*, 60, Commencement Address, box 53, Francis papers, Bentley Library, 61.

71. Quoted in Brandt, "Duplicity," 783. See also Thomas Francis, Jr., "Approaches to Control of Poliomyelitis by Immunological Methods," *Bulletin of the New York Academy of Medicine* 31 (1955): 259–74. On some later criticisms of the design of the trial, see Paul Meier, "Polio Trial: An Early Efficient Clinical Trial," *Statistics in Medicine* 9 (1990): 13–16.

72. Carter, *Breakthrough*, 238. See also Paul, *History of Polio*, 426, and Smith, *Patenting the Sun*.

73. Thomas Francis, Jr., "Approaches to the Prevention of Polio," October 5, 1954, to American Academy of Pediatrics, Chicago, box 53, Francis papers, Bentley Library. This speech was published in the *University of Michigan Medical Bulletin* 22 (1958): 433–45.

74. Rogers, *Dirt and Disease*.

killed virus. "Live virus vaccine has too many potential difficulties and hazards," he told *Modern Medicine* in a featured interview in 1963. "After these many years, vaccinia still carries the risk of secondary damage, such as encephalitis. Purified antigens can have a broader scope, with no interference, no reversions, no complications from unidentified viruses."[75]

The trials established Francis as well as Salk as public figures. Francis, now a national leader in both virology and epidemiology, turned his attention to other projects during the 1950s and 1960s. Within the scientific and popular communities, however, polio remained the major symbol of his life's work. Francis's efforts to turn the focus of epidemiology beyond the investigation of infectious epidemic diseases was reinforced by broader cultural changes, such as the dramatic postwar successes of penicillin and other antibiotics. Many American physicians and lay commentators began to suggest that the medical victory over polio meant that the last great epidemic disease had been conquered. Health officials now turned their attention to the rising importance of endemic diseases such as cancer and heart disease as causes of American mortality.

In the late 1950s, Francis gained support for his interest in studying the epidemiology of endemic, noninfectious disease, and was able to develop the first large-scale community study, involving 9,500 residents of Tecumseh, Michigan, a city twenty-seven miles southwest of Ann Arbor. The Tecumseh project became an integral part of his department's teaching program.[76] Initially designed to explore the early signs of heart disease, the study was quickly expanded to include arthritis, diabetes, chronic pulmonary disease, and other health problems, and gained financial support from the National Institutes of Health. The Tecumseh project, Francis commented in 1963, "brings the principles of infectious disease research into studies of chronic disease."[77] Never loath to confront controversial topics, Francis also urged extensive epidemiological research in dealing with

75. Manuscript of Francis interview, Wendell Weed [Editorial Department, *Modern Medicine*] to Francis, March 7, 1963, box 11, Francis papers, Bentley Library.

76. Frederick H. Epstein, Norman S. Hayner, Benjamin C. Johnson, Henry J. Montoye, and Betty M. Ullman, "The Tecumseh Study: Design, Progress, and Perspectives," *Archives of Environmental Health* 21 (1970): 402–7.

77. Francis, *Modern Medicine* interview, Weed to Francis.

broad public health problems such as the efficacy of fluoride for healthy teeth, and the role of smoking in cancer.[78]

In the last two decades of his life, Francis published reflective pieces on epidemiology and its place in medical research and training. He felt frustrated that many medical teaching programs continued to privilege the laboratory bench and the bedside over the possible insights of field research. The continuing strength of this view reflected the increasing conservatism of organized medicine, which campaigned fervently and successfully in the 1940s and 1950s against proposed health insurance plans, and believed that public health clinics were dangerous to the future of their practice, just as many dentists resisted mass fluoridation. Francis vainly urged medical schools to incorporate what he called the epidemiological approach to medicine. "The study of illness in the patient offers . . . but a limited view of disease as a natural phenomenon," he wrote in 1957. "Disease in the patient represents rather the end result of a process whose origins lie in a complex set of contributory circumstances earlier, often much earlier, while the subject was still a normal member of his community."[79] Epidemiology, Francis argued, could "extend the boundaries of medical research so that the patient is viewed as part of a group or community in which the disorder is arising."[80] In fact, Francis envisioned a world in which the epidemiologist directed the attention and efforts of medical research, bringing to bear "the investigative power of laboratory procedures" and applying them "to the problem at the community level."[81] Francis urged clinicians to concentrate on disease prevention rather than cure. "Epidemiology, by its ability to detect and explain pathogenic relationships, is essential to research and public health, if their function is to maintain health," he argued in 1958. "It is here that epidemiology must direct the attention of medical research and will probably need to take the lead."[82]

---

78. Thomas Francis, Jr., "Epidemiology and the Future of Medicine," 61–63. He also developed a theory of antigenic shifts he called "the doctrine of original sin," which argued that scientists could trace the history of infection in past communities by the reaction to infection in the blood of present generations. Thomas Francis, Jr., "On the Doctrine of Original Antigenic Sin," *Proceedings of the American Philosophical Society* 104 (1960): 573–78.

79. Francis, "Epidemiology and the Future of Medicine," 61.

80. Francis, "What is the Place?" 2.

81. Ibid., 6.

82. Francis, "The Expanding Role of Epidemiology, " 1, 3.

Despite this public rhetoric, Francis acknowledged that the epi-demiological approach continued to remain on the margins of most medical research and training. Students of clinical medicine, he wrote in private to Yale epidemiologist and historian John. R. Paul, should be taught to embrace the "broader point of view of illness as a com-munity problem and its impact upon the population," so that physi-cians "can properly and intelligently guide public health or medicine through the constantly changing social state." Epidemiology should be an important part of the medical school curriculum, not just in a single course but as an attitude that pervades the entire faculty.[83] Yet the "average medical individualist," he admitted, is disdainful of this public health approach, and does not "look to participation or spe-cialization in public health activities with the same reasonableness as to other branches."[84] These views also became part of his public voice. "Most medical students," he told a group of medical educators in 1953, "have not developed through prior experience or education a view of community which permits ready mental excursion into the area of medical ecology."[85] Preventive medicine, he wrote in the *Jour-nal of the American Medical Association* in 1960, "is essentially a ne-glected field."[86]

Francis maintained a deep commitment to research, even though his role in later years was increasingly that of a senior scholar and administrator. He often felt frustrated when his research took third place to his administrative and teaching responsibilities. As early as 1942, Francis complained to a former colleague in New York that,

> At the moment my state of mind is lousy and I would not care to express an opinion on anything of moment. I still seem to be struggling for an opportunity to work and to do what I consider something educational. It would be so easy to decide that one's entire time could be spent in teaching and let the investigative work be philosophical. Perhaps I am doomed not to do any more

83. Francis to John R. Paul [New Haven Hospital], July 8, 1944, box 2-71-C, Francis papers, Bentley Library. Francis argued that interns and residents needed to be trained beyond the individual case, to see that "the hospital is but one of a number of agencies, not just a group of beds, and the patient is a member of a community."

84. Francis to Paul, ibid.

85. Francis, "The Teaching of Epidemiology," 635.

86. Thomas Francis, Jr., "Research in Preventive Medicine," *JAMA* 172 (1960): 998.

research. If so, I may as well die quickly instead of living unhappily and grousing so much.[87]

His last years were spent preparing for a retirement he did not have the opportunity to enjoy, for he died a few months after his formal retirement from the University. In a letter written to Francis's widow Dorothy, Nobel Prize-winning virologist John Enders wrote, "I shall miss Tommy not only because he was always a good friend but also because he set before all of us an example of what a good scientist and physician should be. He was always honest, fair, just and objective."[88] At the memorial service, virologist Colin M. MacLeod commented that Francis was "ambitious, but had such confidence in his own ability to do what needed to be done that he did not feel threatened by others." When people first met Francis, MacLeod remarked, they "thought him prickly and difficult. He persisted in asking the tough scientific questions when almost everyone else was sparring about procedures and administrative arrangements and other matters not central to the issues of the day—the shadows but not the substance."[89]

In 1970 the University of Michigan honored the memory of Francis with the presentation of a formal portrait, and many of his colleagues and friends used the occasion as an opportunity to reflect on his significance in American medicine. Later, the main building of the School of Public Health was named after Francis. Myron E. Wegman, the new dean of the School of Public Health, stressed Francis's "sense of breadth, the all encompassing interest, the curiosity which was indeed insatiable," his "spirit which truly moved mountains." Wegman reminded his Michigan audience that Francis had many interests beyond science, including art, music, and Michigan athletics teams. He was, Wegman commented, a "true scientist, investigator and innovator."[90] In a memorial volume published the same year, Jonas Salk entitled his comments "The Restless Spirit of Thomas Francis,"

---

87. Francis to Dr. Elaine Ralli [New York University College of Medicine], February 16, 1942, box 2, Francis papers, Bentley Library.

88. John Enders to Dorothy Francis, October 2, 1969, box 89, Francis papers, Bentley Library.

89. Colin M. MacLeod, "Thomas Francis, Jr., M.D., 1900–1969," *Archives of Environmental Health* 21 (1970): 228.

90. Wegman, "Francis—An Appreciation," 1–2, 5.

arguing that "the influence of his own boldness continues to live in those whose careers he helped to shape and who shared his commitment to the scientific ideal of the search for, and the exposure of, the truth in nature."[91]

His colleagues and friends consistently described Francis as the epitome of a scientific investigator. But Francis sought to stretch the boundaries of scientific research. He established epidemiology as an activist interdisciplinary field, using the methods of clinical and virological investigation. He was the architect of controlled clinical trials, and established scientifically convincing ways to test the efficacy of vaccines against influenza and polio.

However, the professional and intellectual gaps between research at the bedside, in the laboratory, and in the field, were not resolved by Francis's efforts. As he came to recognize the marginal position of the research epidemiologist, Francis grew somewhat more defensive, as the pedagogical tone of his last years' speeches suggest. His vision draws greater power in retrospect than in its day. After Francis's death, Jonas Salk commented that "Dr. Francis was probably the most important influence in my life."[92] Most of the medical history books do not tell the story this way. But in influenza and polio research in particular, and for the history of public health and medicine in general, Francis stood at the crossroads of virology, immunology, and epidemiology, and provided an expansive vision that stretched from the bench to the field.

91. Salk, "Restless Spirit," 275.
92. Salk, quoted in *Detroit Free Press*, October 2, 1960: "He shaped my career."

Contributors

Joel D. Howell, Associate Professor, Department of Internal Medicine, Department of History, and Department of Health Services Management and Policy, University of Michigan

Kenneth M. Ludmerer, Professor of Internal Medicine and of History, Washington University

Horace W. Davenport, William Beaumont Professor Emeritus of Physiology, University of Michigan

W. Bruce Fye, Chairman, Cardiology Department, Marshfield Clinic, and Adjunct Associate Professor of History of Medicine, University of Washington

Steven C. Martin, Assistant Professor, Department of Epidemiology and Social Medicine and Department of Internal Medicine, Albert Einstein College of Medicine

Steven J. Peitzman, Professor, Department of Internal Medicine, and Associate Professor of Community and Preventive Medicine, Medical College of Pennsylvania

Alexander Leaf, Jackson Professor of Clinical Medicine, Emeritus, Harvard Medical School, and Distinguished Physician, West Roxbury VA Medical Center

Naomi Rogers, Senior Lecturer, Monash University

Index